"In her splendid book, *Unlocking Parental Intelligence*, Dr. Hollman showed parents how to find the meaning in their child's or teen's behavior by reflecting on the child's thoughts and feelings, which may well be different from their own thoughts and feelings about the situation. Finding the meaning underlying the behavior helps parents respond sensitively and supportively. Dr. Hollman's new book gives a concise account of these techniques and, with the aid of helpful real-life examples, shows how to use them to solve problems of exhaustion in children and teens. An excellent resource!"

—JANET WILDE ASTINGTON, PHD

Professor Emeritus, Institute of Child Psychology, University of Toronto; Editor, *Minds in the Making*

"Dr. Laurie Hollman's impressive credentials include three decades as a psychoanalyst doing psychotherapy with children and adults, as well as being a mother and grandmother herself. She has presented us with another in her series of books with advice for busy parents about common and compelling problems with their children.

In this book, she addresses the important problem of exhaustion (i.e., the many varieties of sleep problems which afflict young people). Her thesis is that the Parental Intelligence method, which she again describes here, gives parents a systematic way to discover the often-elusive underlying conflicts which fuel these problems. Without this understanding, finding solutions is harder, if not impossible. She shows us in concise, easy-to-read language how to identify these problems and then offers ideas about how to address them with clarifying clinical examples. Her method promotes a working dialogue and mutual understanding between parents and their children which I believe extends beyond the resolution of the problem at hand. This is a worthwhile read for any parent or anyone who works with children, and I highly recommend it."

—BARBARA G. DEUTSCH, MD

Certified in Psychiatry, American Board of Psychiatry and Neurology, Adult and Child Psychiatry; Certified in Psychoanalysis, American Psychoanalytic Association, Adult and Child Psychiatry

"Please read this book!

Dr. Laurie Hollman has once again given us the gift of her caring, insightful, and practical methods to help us all in our efforts to raise our children (from infancy to the late teen years) and improve all of our relationships in our personal and professional lives.

Dr. Hollman clearly explains the methods which can help all parents (and therapists) develop thoughtful, empathic channels of communication which will allow for parents and children to discover the meaning of their particular disturbance.

By following the steps of Parental Intelligence and not acting impulsively, parents can help themselves and their children find the meaning behind the immediate problems associated with the impact of exhaustion on children and teenagers lives and then work together to solve the problems that become clarified in their discussions.

Through a series of easily understood explanations of exhaustion and the creative use of anecdotes to clearly illustrate the principles involved, Dr. Hollman takes the reader on a journey which illuminates the pathway to enhanced understanding and compassion for our dearest partners and children.

Please read this book!!! It can make a profound addition to your life."

—ERNEST KOVACS, MD, FAPA

Associate Clinical Professor of Psychiatry, Albert Einstein College of Medicine; Supervisor for Marital and Family Psychotherapy, Zucker Hillside Hospital Northwell Health

"Dr. Hollman has done it again! Contained in this handy guide is practical information along with insightful case studies and sound advice regarding the negative psychological effects of sleep deprivation on children and adolescents and what to do about it. Along with the utilization of Dr. Hollman's Parental Intelligence model (*Unlocking Parental Intelligence: Finding Meaning in Your Child's Behavior*), parents are guided in identifying and alleviating the causes of child and adolescent exhaustion. Dr. Hollman does an excellent job of pointing toward wiser parenting choices that alleviate the stressors causing sleep deprivation and forge stronger, more meaningful family bonds."

—LYNN SESKIN, PSYD

Clinical Psychologist; Behavioral Medicine Associates of New York; Behavioral Medicine of Pennsylvania

"Children's exhaustion is a neglected yet vitally important issue with implications for many aspects of their lives. Dr. Hollman illustrates how her approach to parenting can be applied to this issue in order to improve the lives of children and their families."

—JEREMY CARPENDALE, PHD

Professor of Developmental Psychology, Department of Psychology, Simon Fraser University

OTHER BOOKS BY
LAURIE HOLLMAN, PHD

Unlocking Parental Intelligence: Finding Meaning in Your Child's Behavior (Familius, 2015)

The Busy Parent's Guide to Managing Anxiety in Children and Teens: The Parental Intelligence Way (Familius, 2018)

The Busy Parent's Guide to Managing Anger in Children and Teens: The Parental Intelligence Way (Familius, 2018)

The Busy Parent's Guide to Managing Technology with Children and Teens: The Parental Intelligence Way (Familius, 2020)

Are You Living with a Narcissist? How Narcissistic Men Impact Your Happiness, How to Identify Them, and How to Avoid Raising One (Familius, 2020)

The

BUSY PARENT'S
GUIDE to MANAGING

EXHAUSTION

IN CHILDREN AND TEENS

Published by Familius LLC, www.familius.com
1254 Commerce Way, Sanger, CA 93657

Familius books are available at special discounts for bulk purchases, whether
for sales promotions or for family or corporate use. For more information,
contact Familius Sales at 559-876-2170 or email orders@familius.com.

Library of Congress Control Number
2020936500

Print ISBN 9781641702430
Ebook ISBN 9781641703130

Printed in the United States of America

Edited by Kaylee Mason, Sue Franco, and Alison Strobel
Cover design by Carlos Guerrero
Book design by Ashlin Awerkamp

10 9 8 7 6 5 4 3 2 1
First Edition

The
BUSY PARENT'S
GUIDE to MANAGING
EXHAUSTION
IN CHILDREN AND TEENS

THE PARENTAL INTELLIGENCE WAY

LAURIE HOLLMAN, PhD

To Jeff, for his loving compassion and empathy as a husband and father.

ACKNOWLEDGMENTS

I am grateful to three generations of those who have inspired and helped me with this book. I must begin with my husband, Jeff, whose talented writing and editorial skills along with his empathy for children have always strengthened my resolve to put my ideas into words.

In the next generation goes my gratitude to my older son, David, who was raised with Parental Intelligence. I watch David as a father and Claire as a mother carrying out Parental Intelligence with their school-age sons. Both discussed parenting with me, clarifying my ideas. Observing their empathy as parents gives me lasting joy.

My appreciation further extends to my younger son, Rich, also raised with Parental Intelligence. Rich as a father and Shelley as a mother are wonderful examples of parents using loving Parental Intelligence with their daughter. Discussing babyhood with them also clarified my ideas with regard to how Parental Intelligence works so well even during a baby's first year.

Working with the Familius team is always gratifying. I appreciate the publisher, Christopher Robbins, for his accessibility and encouragement as I write for Familius. I am fortunate to work with Brooke Jorden, the managing editor at Familius, who introduced me to the talented editor of this book, Kaylee Mason, who meticulously read each word, gave thought to my concepts, and succeeded in her collaborative way to refine my book and bring it to fruition. Her careful attention to detail, her warm spirit, and facility with language were just what I needed.

I can't conclude without thanking the next generation in line. Thank you, Zander (age 12) and Eddie (age 9), my loving grandsons. Hearing their remarkable use of language at such young ages and watching their vibrant spirits always inspire me to keep on writing. They set the best examples of when we *want* to see kids exhausted. When they are exhausted, it is after a day of work and play, carried out with delight for all they accomplished. It is my pleasure to also see to whom they relate with so empathically. When they confide in me their personal thoughts and wishes, I am reminded of the essence of Parental Intelligence: the close bonds it brings between parent and child, grandparent and grandchild. And I must add even little Hazel (9 months), with her naps and nighttime sleeping, sheds light on how babies, when raised with Parental Intelligence, learn to soothe themselves so they get the sleep they need. Bonding with such a wonderful baby as her grandmother, of course, further confirms the wonder of Parental Intelligence.

CONTENTS

INTRODUCTION

*A*fter thirty years of experience as a psychoanalyst doing psychotherapy with children and adults, I've noted how exhausted kids can get. This inspired me to address parents with an exploration of how exhaustion is a major factor in the well-being of their children and teens. Exhaustion is extreme mental or physical fatigue, a form of depletion of resources. Exhaustion also results from enervation, a feeling of being drained of energy or vitality; a weariness and fatigue that occurs when kids feel depleted due to stress. When adults focus on their own stress and lack of sleep, they recognize how exhausted they find themselves, and now it's time to closely consider that the same issue is important for their kids. For example, adults in the United States were reported to have obtained approximately 8 hours of sleep a night in the 1960s, while more recent Gallup polls reported that adults obtained about 7 hours a night in 2005. A huge Finnish study revealed a more modest decline to 7.3 hours a night. About one in five adults believes that there is a difference of more than one hour between the amount of sleep they need and the amount they actually have (Mendelson, W. B., 2017). But, what about our children?

Exhaustion is a topic that has not received enough attention. In this book we will observe what happens when children don't sleep enough by exploring sleep in mental illnesses, such as depression, and in different developmental stages, such as puberty. Sleep has a restorative role that enriches aspects of daytime functioning such as memory, regulation of mood, pain sensitivity, immune function, and appetite. Exhaustion prevents us from obtaining the right amount of sleep necessary to refine memories, which accumulate daily. During sleep, it has been suggested that excessive synapses are trimmed back, taking away unnecessary material and making memories more precise. Further, sleep cleans up the nervous system of wasteful metabolic products. Given these facts, surely parents need to question the amount of sleep their exhausted kids are getting.

Exhaustion due to sleep deprivation, trauma, and excessive stress is a family as well as societal concern. Sleep serves many functions and the amount needed varies in children at different developmental stages. Those exposed to more outdoor light tend to go to bed earlier and have longer sleep durations.

The US Institute of Medicine and Centers for Disease Control and Prevention have noted the connection of inadequate sleep and exhaustion with chronic conditions including hypertension, depression, and obesity. Also, it is not only duration of sleep, but continuity of sleep, timing, the ability to maintain good wakefulness, and a sense of subjective satisfaction with sleep (Mendelson, W. B., 2017) that is essential for children.

Do we recognize how exhausted so many of our children are and the results of this deprivation? The National Sleep Foundation says that 30 percent of preschoolers don't get enough sleep, and a recently released study by the University of Colorado at Boulder found that sleep-deprived young children consume 20 percent more calories than usual (Hollman, 2016, *Pittsburgh Parent Magazine*). Exhaustion due to acute sleep deprivation leads to decreased vigilance and alterations in mood, cognition, and mental and physical health.

Many children live in a state of partial sleep deprivation: exhaustion in adolescence is considered epidemic. This deprivation leads to deficits in their ability to learn, discover and explore their environment, expand their minds, and get along well with others. Sleep deprivation also affects how their bodies chemically process foods they've eaten and how their immune system fights infections.

My five steps of Parental Intelligence are:

1. Stepping Back
2. Self-Reflecting
3. Understanding Your Child's Mind
4. Understanding Your Child's Development
5. Problem Solving

Using these steps, I will elaborate on how busy parents can identify and alleviate the various reasons their kids are exhausted. With these tools, parents address this essential function of sleep that occupies about one third of their children's existence. Even though sleep deprivation and resulting exhaustion is a process that can be measured physiologically, I will address how it can also be understood psychologically—affecting children's productivity and social behavior.

Exhaustion in children and adolescents is widespread. My motivation for writing this book is to heighten parents' awareness of the significance of this phenomenon, so that they will help their children organize their daily lives to improve their general well-being, productivity, and social competence.

In this book, I will discuss and illustrate how exhaustion in children is often inadvertently caused by adults who do not know how many hours of sleep are typically needed by children and teens at different developmental stages. I will discuss the many factors—such as trauma, loss, depression, burnout, and anxiety—in youngsters that interfere with sleep requirements. I will also explore the need for careful scheduling of activities, how the sleep-wake cycle is not in sync with school schedules, how sleep disturbances and disorders in troubled kids are manifested, and the importance of downtime, particularly unstructured play. We will discover how sometimes unwittingly loving parents make goals for their kids that often interfere with their kids' goals for themselves. This results in exhaustion and parent-child/teen discord.

Once busy parents discover that their children and teens are suffering with exhaustion, parents need to learn the individual meanings behind this problem. With Parental Intelligence can come understanding of the meaning behind our children's exhaustion—which is as varied as our children are.

Using the tools of the Parental Intelligence Way, parents can understand what is going through their child or teen's mind and then collaborate with them to help with their exhaustion and improve their related behaviors. This will not only relieve their sleep debt but also strengthen the parent-child bond.

Different youngsters with a wide range of needs, beliefs, opinions, imaginings, intentions, and goals may be suffering from exhaustion for a vast array of underlying reasons and problems. These need to be identified by their parents, who with Parental Intelligence become "meaning-makers" empowered to read the thoughts and feelings underlying their child's exhaustion. As my previous books on this subject have revealed (*Unlocking Parental Intelligence: Finding Meaning in Your Child's Behavior*, *The Busy Parent's Guide to Managing Anxiety in Children and Teens: The Parental Intelligence Way*, and *The Busy Parent's Guide to Managing Anger in Children and Teens: The Parental Intelligence Way*), parents across the globe have used Parental Intelligence to not only collaborate with their kids to solve problems but strengthen their relationships and find unsurpassed joy in parenting.

With Parental Intelligence, mothers and fathers learn to listen attentively to their children's needs and goals and collaborate with their kids using their accumulated experiences to meet them. I will bring parents up to date with current knowledge of brain activity during sleep stages, so that parents can understand the sleep cycles that their children need for productive, healthy, happy lives.

I have written fictionalized accounts of children and adolescents dealing with exhaustion. To protect the identities of the children and teens who have been actual patients, I have created composites of real kids who have been affected by exhaustion. Their identifying characteristics have been changed.

These stories demonstrate how exhaustion can be managed and resolved using Parental Intelligence, and the results are a closer parent-child bond and greater overall understanding. Parental Intelligence not only provides busy parents a structured approach to helping exhausted kids, but also provides a vision of hope: an avenue for parents to better understand their children at all ages and developmental levels. Using Parental Intelligence, parents support their exhausted kids as they help them solve their problems and lead loving, satisfying lives.

Time is of the essence if we want our children to be cheerful, happy, loving, accomplished youngsters with parents devoted to their physiological and psychological welfare. Exhaustion in children and adolescents is an individual, familial, and societal issue with a huge amount of research backing it up. In the following pages, I will draw on studies to build awareness of this problem and attempt to solve it for growing youngsters and their devoted parents.

CHAPTER ONE

THE PARENTAL INTELLIGENCE WAY

*Exhaustion carries a message—
it's an invitation for understanding.*

While individual parents all face unique challenges, I have discovered many commonalities that affect their varied situations. To help parents face these challenges effectively, I have developed five powerfully valuable steps that allow every busy parent—no matter how different their circumstances—to find meaning behind their child's exhaustion. Beyond that, parents can intelligently and compassionately resolve any underlying problems.

The five steps to Parental Intelligence elaborated on in *Unlocking Parental Intelligence: Finding Meaning in Your Child's Behavior* (2015) are:

1. Stepping Back
2. Self-Reflecting
3. Understanding Your Child's Mind
4. Understanding Your Child's Development
5. Problem Solving

Together, these five steps provide a road map to help you get to your destination: the place where you understand the meaning behind your child's exhaustion. What was once obscure will become clear. When the meaning or meanings behind the exhaustion are understood, it is much easier to decide the best ways to handle the situation. Although the unfolding steps are described in sequence, it is valuable to go back and forth among them as you unlock your Parental Intelligence. Especially when handling step five, the problem-solving step, it can be helpful to look back at step two, self-reflecting, and step three, understanding your child's mind. As new information comes to light, empathy between you and your child will deepen. Going through the five-step process with your child often uncovers problems that are of greater significance than the original behavior. What had been unspeakable will become known, and a new and stronger alliance will form between you and your child.

While exhaustion and its many faces will be discussed in later chapters, I would like to start with explaining the Parental Intelligence method. Although we haven't delved into exhaustion yet and you may have questions, focus on learning the five steps. Once you understand this, we can better understand and communicate about how to help your exhausted child.

STEP ONE
Stepping Back

A parent's first reaction to a child or teen's exhaustion is often emotional. Without distancing themselves from their emotional response, parents often make rash decisions. These decisions lead to actions they later regret, because they do not achieve the desired results. Responding effectively means starting from the same emotional place. This may be uncomfortable, but making it a priority to step back, tolerate your child's feelings, and gradually shift to a more reasoned response will lead to a better outcome.

Imagine taking a video of your child's extreme fatigue, rewinding it, and playing it back in slow motion to get a more detailed picture of what occurred. This means tracking the exhaustion and giving it a beginning, middle, and end. Thinking this way allows you to recall what happened before the exhaustion—what your child did, what was done to your child, what you did, and how you felt. While having information doesn't mean you know what to do with it, it does set the stage for more enlightened parenting choices in the future.

Stepping back requires opening up your thinking and allowing yourself to experience a wide range of emotions without taking immediate action. After a child acts out due to exhaustion, busy parents sometimes feel anxious, on edge, and restless. Because of this they immediately jump into action to alleviate these feelings. Other times busy parents refrain from acting impulsively but feel a nagging tension that interferes with their ability to see the situation objectively. Such a parent may be stuck in one point of view or focus solely on a specific but incomplete set of details. For example, your six-year-old daughter may collapse in a chair at the kitchen table, only to put her head down to rest, not starting her homework. You may sternly tell her to get started on her work, without understanding her fatigue and the reasons for it. It would be better to step back and wait and think about what may be occurring before your worried eyes.

It is not always enough to replay an event, because the replay may confirm or intensify the original emotion. For stepping back to be effective, a busy parent must replay the event while also trying to understand the original emotions the event provoked in him or her.

The process of stepping back also includes the suspension of judgment. This allows you to take time to figure out what happened before taking action. If you never pause, you never allow your emotions to subside and thinking to begin. Stepping back prepares you to engage in the parenting mind-set that says what happened is meaningful. Even in an emergency, once the immediate situation has been handled, there is room for refraining from ready conclusions and for stepping back. Some people primarily look inward and tend to think things through. But not all thinking is productive reasoning; without sufficient information, your thoughts might well be going in circles. Other people primarily look outward and focus on what is going on around them—excluding their own and their child's inner feelings and thoughts when they are trying to understand their child's exhaustion. There may be a reluctance to go inside oneself to experience emotions, for fear of feeling out of control. In both outward- and inward-looking parents, there may be a reluctance to review and rethink their original reaction for fear of appearing soft or inadequate or inconsistent.

Stepping back requires slowing down and thinking about what just happened and how you feel about it, suspending not only judgment of your child's behavior but also of your parenting behavior.

Stepping back gives the parent permission to not always know what to do. Consequently, when a parent reacts one way on the spot but later understands what happened more fully, she can feel confident returning to the child with new thoughts and feelings. These thoughts, once restricted, have begun to expand and offer a new perspective.

When you step back, you prepare yourself to recognize that behaviors have many causes. By pausing when you see the exhausted behavior, you give yourself time to compare the last time the behavior happened to the present situation. You may discover a pattern in your interaction with your child and begin to wonder, Are there any causes for the exhaustion that I couldn't consider last time? You may then begin to see your child's behavior in its many aspects: What triggered the behavior? How long did it last? When did it escalate or decrease? You may also begin to see facets of the exhaustion—facets you were once blind to because of the high emotional states during the incident. Once you are focused on seeking a full knowledge of what happened, you will begin to discover that several problems might be involved in your child's exhaustion. Once you calm down, you begin to notice expressions on your child's face, the words your child said, your child's gestures and postures, and your child's mood and shifts in feelings. After a while, this one behavior—exhaustion (mental or physical fatigue)—can be broken down and understood as many separate behaviors. We will address these separate behavior possibilities in the chapters that follow.

Stepping back can open up your mind to such an extent that you may feel that you're observing a different behavior or group of behaviors than what you did originally. For example, you may first think that your eight-year-old child's angry outburst is because he failed his math test. However, after stepping back you realize that he is exhausted from staying up too late studying to no avail and so he is very irritable.

Stepping back gives you the space and time to evaluate the situation, examine and question assumptions, and realize that the situation isn't fully understood.

Take as much time as you need to consider what is happening. In your mind, say to yourself, *Slo-o-o-w down. Take your time. Hold on. Don't thrust forward.*

Resist those impulses. Breathe deeply. Sit quietly. Consider what to say or do, if anything.

Both mothers and fathers who are invested in the *process*—not just the outcomes—of child rearing have a greater tendency to naturally step back. Fathers and mothers can encourage and help each other in stepping back, particularly in two-parent households where co-parenting is a goal. Parents who live in separate residences but share in co-parenting can also help each other to step back. They can find good alternatives to impulsive reactions as they learn how to balance their responsibilities for both work and childcare—and then share their insights with each other. The significance of mothers and fathers supporting each other in the process of stepping back cannot be underestimated. A mother may be the buffer to a father's automatic release of anger, just as he may do the same for her.

When you give yourself permission to slow down before reacting and deciding on consequences, you can reduce stress and feel more in control. Stepping back changes the tone between parent and child. When children see their parents taking their time, they start to feel—perhaps cautiously at first—that their parents can be trusted to guide them.

Summary of Stepping Back

The purpose of stepping back is to set the stage for parents to take stock of their feelings and organize their thinking about the exhaustion behavior that has just occurred or is occurring. This is just common sense, but it requires tolerating frustration—a skill we are hoping to also teach our children. While thinking over what occurred, parents ideally suspend judgment and acknowledge that exhaustion carries meaning. This first step in the Parental Intelligence parenting approach helps parents to embrace the concept that fatigue communicates a child's feelings and motives and may indicate problems that need to be solved in the parent-child relationship.

The next step, self-reflecting, increases a parent's ability to understand *his* feelings, motives, and actions following what he thought was simply an instance of his child's exhaustion.

STEP TWO
Self-Reflecting

Self-reflecting allows you to discover how your past affects your present approach to parenting or how something on your mind that has to do with your current situation is interfering with your ability to listen to your child attentively. Self-reflecting allows you to observe yourself objectively and think about the genesis of your feelings, motives, and actions in both present and previous relationships. This step requires honestly questioning why you behaved the way you did. Sounds logical, but it can be hard. It's so tempting to just jump to ready solutions and skip questioning what's going on inside of you.

For parents, self-reflecting is an extension of stepping back. It requires you to consider what led to your specific responses to your child's exhaustion, prompts you to think about your actions from many perspectives, and allows you to consider many causes for your responses. That sounds like a tall order, but if you take it bit by bit, you will be amazed at what you discover. Self-reflecting happens after the incident of your child's exhaustion—maybe hours or days later. Sometimes it is subtle. You may be in your car at a red light, and your mind returns to the situation. By considering your reactions, you may suddenly see them from a different perspective. You discuss the situation—and specifically your reactions—with a friend or a spouse, and they offer new perspectives on your reactions. Other times you may purposefully rethink the exhausted behavior and ask yourself if there are other ways to approach the situation or if you could mirror the ways you've seen other parents react to similar situations. You begin to question, *Why did I react that particular way?* or *What were my motives and intentions?* or *What in my past affected my thinking and actions in the present?* or *What were my emotional reactions to my child's behavior, and where did they come from?*

If you allow yourself to take time to self-reflect, it isn't as difficult as you might imagine. In fact, you may notice that you feel more confident as you strive to look inward. Self-reflecting is a discovery process. You are getting to know yourself better. It feels good. Self-reflecting allows you to learn more about yourself as a child and teenager and about the effect your experiences may have on your present reactions to your child.

Self-reflecting often leads to the realization that you take your child's fatigue very personally. That's hard to accept, but it's also relieving to understand. Have you ever found yourself angrier than a situation warranted and caught yourself midstream before bursting out with fury? With some quick thinking, you may realize that what's making you angry has something to do with yourself—not your child. Then you reflect further and consider how to be authoritative, yet kind and compassionately involved in your child's life. This takes a strong sense of self—a capacity for self-awareness.

Practicing this self-awareness can help you to feel better about yourself.

Your relationships with your own caregivers—which may include parents, teachers, and other adults—during infancy, childhood, and adolescence may determine your capacity for reflective functioning as an adult. Your early experiences shape the expectations of future attachments. When you strive to bring your own conflicts from the past to the forefront of your mind and understand them, it can help you to help your child. Admittedly, patterns of relationships are often unconscious and difficult to change without therapeutic intervention. Nonetheless, even if parents seek treatment, they can't just wait for their therapy to end before helping their child; their child continues to grow and needs help now. It can be surprisingly effective for parents to realize that their thoughts and reactions can come from the past and may affect the specific behavior in question.

Think of a distressing behavior your child exhibits and consider your feelings during the incident. Now go back and find a past experience that triggered the same or similar feelings. Review the experience slowly, like a story, in as much detail as you can. Think about the people in your life at that time and what they meant to you, then and now. You may find that your child's present behavior triggers aspects from that past situation.

Ask yourself some questions: *Does my child's behavior remind me of my behavior in the past? Does my child's behavior remind me of someone else's behavior in the past? Was my past situation a marker for me in some way? Was the past situation a turning point in my life? Do I have unresolved feelings about that time?* As you go through this mental and emotional process, you may begin remembering more and more. Thoughts and details that were hidden for years begin to surface. All of these memories may very well have to do with the way you now react to your child.

For example, you might remember being your child's age and feeling exhausted all the time. It may even surprise you to realize this. In your case, you were exhausted because you didn't have a set bedtime routine and your parents weren't aware that rituals for sleeping well matter. You know this isn't the case for your seven-year-old, so something else is amiss. You realize you need to reflect; this will help you to figure out the meaning behind your child's exhaustion. It may look like yours was but is actually different. There are several possibilities. If your child's behavior, manner, posture, or tone of voice resonates with how you interacted with someone else at earlier times in your life, you may be reacting to your child the way you reacted when you were younger. This can be very enlightening to discover. Or you may be reacting to your child the way you wished you had reacted when you were younger. Have you had any epiphanies? Are light bulbs going off? If your mind is racing backward, you may be feeling much more in touch with your reactions. Alternatively, your reaction to your child's behavior may be occurring because someone once reacted to you the way your child is behaving now. This may be very upsetting to you. As past and present have converged, it's no wonder you react so strongly.

Your capacity for self-reflection may grow as your child grows. If your child reaches an age that was troublesome for you when you were young, conflict between you and your child may ensue because you are reminded of your unresolved problems at that age. However, realizing that you dealt with similar issues can open up your understanding by leaps and bounds. It may take a lifetime to become adept at self-reflecting, but as you're learning, you can improve your relationship with your child.

There are many past stereotypes about women being more empathic and tuned-in to feelings than men are, which you might think would affect a man's capacity to self-reflect. However, in thirty years of experience with many different parents, I have not seen either gender prefer self-reflecting more than the other. I have, however, found that men's past experiences with their fathers when they were children affect what they expect of themselves as fathers. Men either want to give their children the same positive experiences they had with their fathers, or they want to give their children better fathering experiences than they had. Both women and men whose fathers were not active in their lives may have low expectations for the father's involvement with their children.

Women with such low expectations may be surprised and pleased when their children's fathers want to be invested in parenting. Or, this may have been part of what attracted them to these men. Women may look back at their mothers' involvement with them as something they want to emulate or change when they become mothers. When parents engage in this kind of self-reflecting, these yearnings come to light and can have a positive effect on their children. All of this can come to light after self-reflection and can help busy parents to notice their own reactions to a child's behavior.

Summary of Self-Reflecting

As parents understand themselves better through self-reflecting, they become more consciously aware of the impact their past or current problems have on their present responses to their children in specific situations.

As a result, negative, fast reactions can recede into the background, while you can discover alternative reactions that are far more effective at handling a specific situation. Parental self-reflecting leads to new levels of compassion and resilience in parent-child relationships. Stepping back and self-reflecting add great depth to understanding your current reactions to your child.

Self-reflecting helps mothers and fathers question why they react quickly instead of searching for meaning. In time, parental impulsive reactions wane, creating a readiness for flexible, sensitized decision-making. Insightful decision-making builds a bridge to your child that leads to understanding your child's mind—step three in this parenting approach.

STEP THREE
Understanding Your Child's Mind

"What's on your mind?" is a question often asked casually, but understanding your child's mind is central to knowing your child. This casual question prompts a series of other questions about parenting that carry important answers. Does understanding the mind of your child help your child cope? Does understanding the mind of your child help you cope? And what roles do emotions play in your child's thinking?

Understanding your child's mind starts with knowing your child's mental states. What are they? The term *mental state* refers to all mental experiences. A short list of mental states would include intentions, thoughts, desires, wishes, beliefs, and feelings. Additionally, it's important to understand that contradictory and diverse mental states can occur at the same time. For example, a teen wishes (a mental state) to have ice cream, and yet he feels he shouldn't because he intends (a mental state) to lose weight so he can make the wrestling team.

When I talk about mental states, I am also referring to physical states, because they are inextricably interwoven. This can be especially seen in adolescence. A teen has a mind with feelings and desires. How does the attentive mother notice these mental states? When a teen feels self-doubt (a mental state), he may withdraw to his room. The mother knows not to chase after him and then observes contentment (another mental state) when the teen reappears and wants to chat. Your ability as the parent to understand your child's mind is directly related to your ability to self-reflect. As described above, self-reflecting is your capacity to think about your own past experiences. Self-awareness and your awareness of the mental states of others are closely linked. When, with self-reflecting, you are able to understand how your own mind is working, it becomes easier to realize that your child's mind is separate and autonomous from yours. However, if you do not self-reflect and understand this, you may attribute your own mental states (intentions and feelings) to your child and her behaviors.

For example, let's say you are angry at your ten-year-old for being curt with you. It's breakfast time, and you laid out a balanced, delicious meal for him on the kitchen table: toast with his favorite jam, granola, and his favorite fruit-juice smoothie—the works! However, he barely says "good morning," grabs a piece of toast, and runs out the door. You feel disrespected. He barely noticed what you'd done and you're angry he wasn't grateful for the lovely meal you prepared. You then assume he was mad at you from the quick, "See ya," he called without even looking at you. His anger was completely unjustified and the assumption is simple: you're angry; he's angry. You've forgotten that your child's feelings and intentions may be quite different from your own. In this example, your child may have simply been curt because he was exhausted and running late for the school bus. He was in a hurry and wasn't mad at you at all.

Here's another example. A child is frustrated when the dinner in a restaurant isn't served quickly and complains vigorously that she's starving. She keeps looking at her phone and writing texts to her friends to distract herself from her hunger. She's starving because she is exhausted—which only makes her hungrier. Her father, however, had a big lunch, is enjoying everyone's company, and doesn't mind waiting. He finds his fifteen-year-old daughter's complaints rude and scolds her, telling her to quiet down and put away her phone or she can't go out later. The daughter feels resentful. The father's and daughter's mental states—their intentions and feelings—are different. This girl's father mistakenly assumed that what is on his mind is also on his daughter's mind. He falsely made the assumption that she was enjoying everyone's company and didn't mind waiting when she was immersed in just feeling hungry so couldn't even focus on the conversation.

An inability to be aware that your own mental state is different from that of your child can lead to misinterpretation of the intent of your child's behavior. This causes a rupture in your parent-child relationship and, sometimes, unnecessary punishment. Understanding your child's mind depends on realizing the links between intentions, feelings, thoughts, and behaviors, and looking for meanings behind behaviors. Behaviors and feelings are inextricably bound together.

For instance, a mother might say to her son, "You punched the wall when your brother interrupted your video game. He's been doing this for weeks, and your exhaustion, and thus frustration, has reached its limit. Think about it. I bet by hitting the wall, you were avoiding hitting him." Now that she's planted a new idea in her son's mind, she continues, "Let's think and talk more about your exhaustion, so you don't ever need to punch a wall." She's now connected his emotional state—frustration due to exhaustion—to his behavior—punching.

Busy parents who approach situations like this mother are attuned to what's going on in their child's mind and, in turn, what caused the behavior. While the father in the example at the restaurant was unable to shift from a punitive stance to understanding his child's mind, this mother links her son's internal emotional state to his exhaustion.

Most parents and children can recognize each other's moods but need time to figure out the reasons behind a particular mood. Behavior is meaningful, even if you don't catch on right away. Often, you need to let the behavior sit in your mind and wait for its meaning to emerge. This is stepping back. If, as a busy parent, you know your child very well and have been trying to understand his or her mind for many years and over many developmental stages, you can become quite an expert at reading your child's moods and thoughts.

Of course, it's important to check your ideas with your child. This shows empathy: "It seems like your teacher hurt your feelings, so you bolted out of the classroom. Was it something like that?" Let's say your child then reveals that she is feeling hurt. After hearing your child's response, you might continue: "Now that we figured out what was going on in your mind, were there other choices you may have had that would be a better way to react the next time you feel hurt?"

No one likes being instructed on how they should feel, but it sure feels good to be understood. Everyone appreciates empathy, and feeling understood can help a child contain his emotions and begin to think them through. When a child feels that his parent understands what is going on inside his mind, he feels attended to and supported, and then can think further about how to handle situations.

It's important to realize, however, that all parents had experiences growing up that caused the formation of emotional triggers that still exist in the present—often unconsciously. These triggers prompt responses to their children's behaviors, and they are very hard to unlearn. This can interfere with empathy. Thus, early emotional triggers in the parent may lead to misinterpretations of what is actually leading to their child's exhaustion. This can be resolved by returning to further self-reflecting and then empathy can resume.

What does understanding your child's mind have to do with empathy? Understanding your child's mind is part of empathy—understanding the emotional states of another person. For example, parents form an idea of what their child might be feeling when they see a particular emotional expression on her face. It's like trying to step into your child's shoes and see from her point of view.

Understanding your child's mind in this way is a creative act. However, it is an act of imagination with severe limitations: no one can know another person's mind with complete accuracy. Thus, it is best to approach the task by asking questions rather than by making statements. This empathic approach can be difficult if you did not have parents who modeled empathy. If you had caretakers in your life who didn't empathize with your needs and emotions and who didn't explore how people's behaviors impacted others, empathizing with your own children will most likely not come naturally. So, give yourself time to catch on to your child's feelings. It's remarkable how good it feels when you understand something new about your child. You know you've done well when your son or daughter says, "Hey, Mommy. You really get it. Thanks."

Empathic parents tend to raise empathic children. They become interested in how their parents think and feel and may be quite good listeners. As your child learns that he can look to you to understand his states of mind (intentions, feelings, beliefs), he may become interested in understanding your states of mind. It's not that roles should be reversed, where the child becomes the listener to the parents' problems, but it does mean that an empathic child will want to understand where his parents (and other people around him) are coming from. In order to understand your child's mind, it helps to be a good observer. Verbal communication is only one piece of the puzzle. Watch your child's facial expressions to get an idea of what's on his mind. For example, maybe your child won't talk to you, but he is constantly rolling his eyes or pursing his lips. He's upset with you because he feels like you're overstepping your boundaries with him about something personal. Although you weren't in tune to this previously, you realize—upon self-reflecting—that maybe he's feeling embarrassed about what you're talking about; and you back down gently.

Sometimes we are blind to an emotion in our children that we block out in ourselves. For instance, an exhausted parent who blocks out hurt is blind to her exhausted child's hurt. Thus, parents can misperceive what they feel, thinking they feel only one mental state (exhaustion) while truly feeling something else (hurt). If this is true, then recognizing your child's hurt behind her exhaustion might lead to you feeling your own. If you don't know what is on your own mind—what you are thinking and feeling—you may subsequently be blocked from understanding what is on your child's mind—what she is thinking and feeling. You may draw erroneous conclusions. It's helpful if you understand that mental states are changeable, that they affect behavior, and that understanding them leads to stronger parent-child relationships.

If both mother and father are involved in their children's daily lives, the diverse interpretations of their parental communications make children feel listened to and understood. The mother or father doesn't always have to immediately catch on to what their child is trying to get across. This takes time. It is the parents' efforts that matter. Children become more confident when both parents value their ideas and feelings. At the same time, parents can discover that their children are more capable than they knew as they learn the meanings behind their kids' behaviors. Mothers and fathers may understand their infants', children's, and teens' minds differently by interpreting behaviors, sounds, words, gestures, facial expressions, and other body language in different ways. However, what matters most is that both parents are interested in what goes on in their child's mind and how their child's mind works. Parental Intelligence highlights the immense importance of this type of maternal and paternal involvement.

Summary of Understanding Your Child's Mind

Trying to understand your child's mind is essential for knowing who he is, how he thinks and feels, and why he may be exhausted. If busy parents want to change their child's behavior, they need to learn about their child's mental states. What is on the parent's mind affects what is on the child's mind—and vice versa. Parents who have their child's mind in mind are more likely to have children who are self-reflective and secure. Parents who are able to think about their children's minds manage their parent-child relationships better and are more effective in resolving inevitable conflicts and arguments.

Trying to understand your children's minds shows them you believe in them and teaches them to believe in themselves. Treating your children like capable human beings with well-functioning minds and good intentions builds trust.

STEP FOUR
Understanding Your Child's Development

There are developmental stages at which children master different skills, but not all children reach those stages at the same time. For example, your seven-year-old may be more adept at completing a math problem than a nine-year-old. Your thirteen-year-old may be more empathic than a sixteen-year-old. Two children in the same grade may perform differently on the same assignment. Have you noticed that when your firstborn was a teen she had great problem-solving skills and a high level of frustration tolerance, while your next-in-line was pretty inflexible and had trouble handling frustration as a teen?

The age when a child reaches a certain skill level is the child's *developmental age* for that skill, regardless of the child's chronological age. When parents take into account the developmental age of their child—which reflects the stage the child has reached in mastering certain capacities—parents and children get along better. What capacities should you look for? Notice your child's interpersonal skills: impulse control, effective communication, and empathy. Other skills include thinking or cognition. Watch for the development of individual capacities such as autonomy and identity formation. You'll probably find your children aren't consistent across the board, but they have strengths and weaknesses. The chronological age may not be the same as the developmental age for any of these capacities, and children may be at different developmental levels for different skills. When you set expectations for your children, be sure they reflect each child's developmental levels, which may fall behind or step ahead of their chronological age.

Once you have taken the earlier steps by stepping back, self-reflecting, and understanding your child's mind, understanding your child's developmental stage becomes essential for effective problem solving. Especially when it comes to exhaustion, as children need different amounts of sleep at different developmental stages. Mothers and fathers should also be aware of their own physical and emotional changes during their child's development that may affect their readiness to understand the stages their child is going through. For example, if a parent is recently unemployed, he may be so concerned with his plight that he fails to be attentive to a child's needs or reactions to a situation.

For many parents, at different times in their parenting life, it may be necessary to return to self-reflection before understanding what to expect of their child at specific stages of development. Then they become confident setting reasonable limits that their child accepts.

Summary of Understanding Your Child's Development

Parents who understand and nurture their child's development can more effectively evaluate what they can expect of their child, especially with regard to sleep behaviors. These behaviors become signals of a child's developmental stage or of a child's need for meaningful communication. For example, your child's sleep behavior may lead you to view him as distressed and in need of help clarifying his motivations and intentions. Rules can be devised, limits can be set, and achievements can be expected that fit your child's developmental age. Consequently, children can comprehend limits, tolerate frustration, be empathic of others, and form rich, enduring parent-child and peer relationships.

STEP FIVE
Problem Solving

The more you continue working on the first four steps, the more natural and effective they will become, getting you ready for the last step—problem solving. Interestingly, after working through the first four steps, the initial problem—the specific behavior, exhaustion—has become part of a set of problems to be solved over time. The immediate importance of the initial behavior may have lessened because it has been recognized as a symptom of more pressing issues lying underneath. These are the problems you ultimately hope to solve, together with your child, using Parental Intelligence. For example, you may have first noticed your child's angry outburst, but then realized it was a reflection of her fatigue that you need to learn the meaning of. This is a more important issue that needs to be tackled first.

The steps in this book that lead to problem solving are based on your desire to have a strong, healthy, and joyful relationship with your child. It is usually possible to repair a relationship, even if it has been ruptured in past conflicts. The key to repairing a ruptured relationship is a secure, trusting relationship. Without a good relationship, problems are rarely solved.

The steps leading from stepping back to problem solving seem linear, but you may need to go back and forth among them. This is truly significant because the earlier steps, or lack thereof, directly affect the process of problem solving. If, for example, you attempt to talk with your child and problem solve, but then the conversation slips back into blaming by either you or your child, it is time to go back to earlier steps. If, as another example, you or your child consider each other's behavior to be intentionally oppositional, authoritarian, or a power struggle, then, again, it is important to go back to earlier steps. Or if, during problem solving, you find that you or your child's voice is tinged with sarcasm, you may be off track; a new problem may have surfaced, signaled by the sarcasm. Address that issue first, and use your new skills (e.g., understanding your child's mind) to identify what is driving your child to speak that way to you. If you find you are becoming sarcastic, angry, or more jittery and irritable than usual, use your new skills (e.g., stepping back) to reflect on potential triggers. In each of these instances, taking a break from problem solving to figure out your own and your child's reactions will be worth the effort.

While problem solving, you may realize you need to be more reflective about your view of reality and your child's view of reality. If, indeed, you and your child can see the problem from each other's point of view, both you and your child should be ready to problem solve together.

Let's think more about points of view. It is worth revisiting self-reflecting at this point. Maybe you suddenly realize that your child's view of an experience is similar to one you held as a child, too. For example, your daughter explains she is bored and falls asleep in social studies class because she honestly dislikes the teacher's attitude. This reminds you of similar feelings you had when you were in eighth grade when you used to act out and get low grades, so you are sympathetic but want your child to do well in school regardless of the teacher's personality. This sudden realization gives you pause and helps you better understand both your child and yourself. You also realize that you were resistant to understanding your daughter in the first place because she provoked the past in you, something you did not want to remember. Re-experiencing past emotions and events can have the benefit of allowing you to rethink the present event. You can then better understand where your child is coming from and solve the problem together. Sometimes the problem that needs to be addressed isn't an event or behavior, but instead is the way you communicate with your child. When you realize your reactions came from the past, your interactions become increasingly empathic. Continuing the above example about the child sleeping through her social studies class because she was turned off by the teacher's attitude, the parent and child may have an insightful discussion about how kids react to adults' moods and then sabotage their own performance. Perhaps, this parent and child could problem solve by getting the disgruntled sleepy child a social studies tutor—after spending time understanding that sleeping was not a good option for tuning out a teacher. With that understanding, the child has more options and a more enlightened view of teachers as adults with varied personalities that needn't interfere with the subject matter. That understanding, plus the tutor, may not only solve the problem at hand but also give the child more understanding of how teachers can affect their levels of achievement. In this instance, the daughter learns she is capable of doing well, and she learns that her reactions to the teacher's style affected her negatively and unnecessarily.

In other words, for problem solving to become possible and effective, you need to try to understand what is on both your mind and your child's mind. You need to view the situation not only from your point of view but also from your child's vantage point. If you can do so and share your understanding with your child, your child will be prompted to reciprocate. If you can't comprehend and picture your child's reality, you can't solve a problem with him.

Your child, too, needs to try to understand your view of the problem. If both of you can't embrace the other's point of view of the problem, you both must sort that out before advancing to solving the problem at hand. Problem solving also needs to take into account your child's developmental stage, which allows you to understand your child's actual capabilities and skill set relevant to the problem.

Communication through speech, gestures, and facial expressions are affected by moods and temperaments. We all know how variable moods can be from moment to moment or day to day. Communication is not always smooth when problem solving; it can be awkward and uncertain. If you and your child expect that there may be many uncomfortable moments, then they won't deter you from continuing to pursue the step of problem solving. Problem solving aims to find mutual meanings, which may be new to both participants. Meanings are exchanged through taking collaborative turns in talking things out in order to correct misinterpretations of the behavior in question.

The benefits are numerous. Both parents and children are more effective as they repair their differences and develop a positive feeling about their relationship with each other. Parent and child learn new coping skills that can be used in the future, which fosters optimism for future interactions. Problem solving takes time, but for busy parents these steps give them a structure they can depend on and come back to when they have more time. Sticking with it and being persistent can be difficult. Also, like any plan, it's only a good one if it is carried out. Remember that it took a long time for the problems between you and your child to build up; it will also take time to repair them. The busy parent can explain that to his child and make a plan for when and how they will find time to problem solve. The challenge is to hold on to your belief that the relationship can be salvaged and the problems can be resolved. Without this commitment, things can fall apart quickly. When your child sees that your commitment is loving and genuine, she will likely feel deeply cared for and persist as well. When both you and your child are determined to use your energy to make problem solving work, it is highly likely that things will work out to everyone's benefit.

The structure of the family has been changing in recent decades. For example, current trends suggest that both mothers and fathers feel conflicted about time spent away from family and struggle to maintain balance between working outside the home—often for very long hours—and spending time with their children. Although either or both parents work outside the home, they spend more time with their children than parents did in the past. This gives mothers and fathers more opportunities to be devoted to carrying out the step of problem solving with their children. For children, problem solving is a developmental process and skill. Reciprocal interactions drive interpersonal development. When you, as the parent, engage in this process, you will find you are developing a collaborative relationship with your child. The ability to do this will rest on the mother-child and father-child relationships that have been growing as you accomplish the earlier steps of Parental Intelligence.

During problem solving, you will engage in a give-and-take between you and your child. Problem solving is a relational process. When children learn that their parents realize the underlying problems behind their original behavior, they may become more open than ever to hearing what their parents have to say. This is because they are feeling understood.

Children are often relieved to know that their mother or father is open to their points of view, wants to hear about their feelings, and is aware of the developmental struggles they may be going through. In turn, as a parent feels the reciprocity of the open dialogue with his child, he slowly relaxes and trusts the open, honest, and empathic communication.

In the best possible world, each parent uses Parental Intelligence and is open to reciprocal communication. If not, problem solving will be most productive only with the parent who has followed the prior steps fully.

Summary of Problem Solving

Problem solving may appear to be the single most important step. To problem solve well, however, the earlier steps are just as—if not more—important. Because without these steps, you may not know what the most essential problems really are.

Parental Intelligence is a relationship-based approach to rearing children as opposed to a punishment-based approach. Parents don't lose their say about their children's behaviors, but rather they understand the reasons behind the behavior, its context, and workable approaches that help their children and themselves to change the behavior or their view of the behavior.

Parents and children alike feel comfortable enough to bring their agendas to the table in the hopes of not only solving the immediate situation, but also being understood. The parents' purpose is not only to find the underlying meaning in the particular behavior, but also to help their child learn to be aware of feelings, engage in logical thinking, face challenging developmental passages, and include the art of discussion in relationships. As parents step back, reflect, understand their own and their children's minds, and learn about child development, the meaning behind behaviors becomes clearer, and the actual overarching problems can be solved. In a secure relationship, where parents and children engage each other in reciprocal ways, and where the concerns of both parent and child are taken into consideration, alternate means to solving problems arise.

In an insecure attachment, where the bonds are more tenuous, problem solving is much more difficult, since parent and child do not reciprocally engage or trust each other. Children may expect that their parents will not be sensitive to their emotional and social cues, and those children will not want to engage in discussions for that very reason. Parents may likewise expect that children will just tune them out and not want to engage in discussions. Therapeutic help may be needed to redress this distrust and shift the relationship into a more secure position. When it is time to problem solve, children and parents may slip into avoidance tactics. They may change the subject, move around, begin a round of keeping secrets, hide their feelings about the relationship, and generally find ways to interrupt the interaction. This is where empathy comes in. Parents may need to clearly point out that their children are avoiding the discussion and that they hope to understand why. Similarly, the behavior that began this process may reappear, demonstrating that the parents may have begun to unintentionally avoid the behavior's underlying problems. Parents also need to take into account that young children don't think or articulate as quickly as adults. Adults, therefore, need to allow for pauses and silences. Parents need to stop themselves from slipping into lectures and coaching before the child has a chance to absorb what is being discussed and let the child have her say. Adolescents, too, need to avoid lecturing their parents with broad "philosophies of life" that drive the conversation from the issues at hand.

In time, if parent and child engage with each other, focus on their relationships, and empathize with each other, and especially if parents make it a priority to identify the meanings behind their child's behaviors, a new quality of interaction will come to life. Problems can and will be solved to mutual satisfaction. When this relationship is well-established, busy parents will likely find that they interact with their kids in more empathic ways and that the element of time is not so much an issue. This is because parents and kids now trust each other to come back when they have more time to completely solve a problem. Having a five-step structure to rely on facilitates quick thinking and immediate or transitional problem resolution when parents and kids are busy and on the run.

SUMMARY
Five Steps to Parental Intelligence

Through the evolving process of unlocking Parental Intelligence, each parent learns a great deal about their own mind and the mind of their child. That is, each parent must accept the challenge of learning what is going on inside himself if he is to discover what is going on inside his exhausted child.

Ruptures in a parent-child relationship cannot be avoided, but the continued experience of repair secures and strengthens the relationship. The child learns to trust the parent because she believes her parent is invested in understanding a vast array of emotions. Respect and trust are earned as pleasures and are shared, and problems are solved.

Different parents will find different steps to be harder or easier to master, depending on the degree of empathy they had already embraced as part of themselves before beginning the process. Each reader who has used the Parental Intelligence approach has learned how to decipher meaning behind child behavior, only to find that there are overarching problems to be unmasked.

Becoming a meaning-maker is a profound experience that can change how you, as a parent, view children and teens and, most fundamentally, yourself. Parents who have unlocked their Parental Intelligence are introspective mothers and fathers who have become willing to understand and take a look at themselves in order to understand their children and know how they think. Parents learn not only what they and their children think about, but also how they carry out the thinking process.

Learning to use Parental Intelligence can offer a new stage of a mother's or father's parenting life that will have lifelong results in how family members engage each other, care for each other, and view and solve problems over the long haul.

As we face the new generations, this collaborative approach becomes even more important than ever before as children expect to be heard, respected for their knowledge, and empathized with. The Parental Intelligence Way fits the bill.

CHAPTER TWO

LEARNING ABOUT THE EXHAUSTED CHILD THE PARENTAL INTELLIGENCE WAY

CAL

Two-year-old Cal is curled up on the couch at five o'clock in the afternoon, sound asleep, when his mother returns from work. It's the second time this week she's discovering him in a deep sleep at this odd time of day. He usually races to greet her when she arrives home from work. She is not only disappointed in missing the warm hello hug but is also concerned and worried that he's oversleeping. Daria, the child-minder whom Cal's mother has come to rely on since she went back to work when Cal was four months old, assures her that Cal has had his nap and played happily during the day; Daria, too, finds this exhaustion bewildering.

Strongly committed to using the five steps of Parental Intelligence, Cal's mother quickly turns to step one, stepping back. This means she pauses without reacting quickly in order to consider the major premise of Parental Intelligence—that a child's behavior has meaning. She attempts to experience her wide range of emotions without taking immediate action. If she didn't pause but rushed to awaken her son without suspending judgment, he might see her panic and become unnecessarily distressed.

Instead she thinks back to the last few days to review Cal's sleep pattern. He has been easily falling asleep at about 7:30 at night after she reads him a bedtime story. He has been awakening at 6:30 when the child-minder arrives, and they share breakfast together, starting off a peaceful day. She's been leaving for work at her usual time, 7:30 a.m., although she realizes now that Cal has been a bit clingy—which is unusual because he adores and loves his child-minder. Cal's father also shares their breakfast and leaves at the same time.

Except for the clinginess, she doesn't think of anything else unusual. She then awakens Cal gently with a warm hug and kiss, and he smiles, returning the hug. Before the child-minder leaves for the day, she notices that Cal gives her kind of a cold shoulder—not the usual good-bye kiss. This stays in Cal's mother's mind, and Daria gives her a look that suggests Daria is concerned, too. That evening, however, Cal goes to sleep as usual, the extra nap not disturbing his routine.

Step two of Parental Intelligence is self-reflecting, which permits Cal's mother to muse about how her past affects her present approach to Cal. Her self-reflection allows her to think about her own past and search for the genesis of her feelings, motives, and actions in both present and previous relationships. When she mentions her concerns about Cal's sleepiness, her husband at first brushes it off, saying sometimes kids just need extra sleep.

However, Cal's father, like his mother, recalls that self-reflecting is a discovery process and looks a little deeper into his feelings. He realizes that he, too, is puzzled by Cal's behavior. However, he knows he is more detached from Cal than his wife is. Originally, he hadn't wanted to adopt a child, but his love for his wife and her needs superseded his reluctance. He carefully admits to her these initial feelings, which leads them to recall Cal's entrance to their family.

Cal was adopted at birth. His biological mother was supposed to give him up immediately but insisted at the last second to hold and feed him, perhaps forming a bond that was deep inside of Cal. Cal's parents always wondered about that. But he bonded with them in the first few months, especially with his mother, and they forgot about that transition until now.

Self-reflecting often leads to thoughts about one's own upbringing, but for Cal's parents this wasn't the case. They both had enough nurturance, which is why they wanted to give the same to their son.

They continued talking and began step three, understanding your child's mind, and proceeded to review more of Cal's birth history. Cal was an easy baby while his mother was on maternity leave, and his father participated more at a distance. When it was time for them to return to work, they were delighted to find the experienced child-minder, Daria. Cal's father had returned to work after a few weeks, but his mother stayed home for the first four months. During the last month of her time at home, Cal's mother shared Cal's care with Daria, so the transition could be as smooth as possible. Cal did show signs of separation distress when his mother first went to work, but then comfortably settled into a soothing routine with Daria.

So, what was going on now in Cal's mind that would lead to the extra afternoon nap? A light bulb went off in Cal's mother's head as she realized that she had not considered the effect on her son when Daria had suddenly announced that she had to leave when Cal turned two. Cal didn't react at first—almost as if he was denying the implications.

Cal's mother now realizes the importance this holds for Cal. It is simply too much for him to absorb. She realizes that Cal is withdrawing from his overwhelming feelings of loss. First, he lost his birth mother, then his adoptive mother goes back to work, and now he is losing Daria—much too much for a two-year-old to process and understand. So, Cal is sleeping away his excess emotions. He is in fact withdrawing from the change he is about to experience.

Turning to step four, understanding your child's development, Cal's parents realize that losing a caretaker is immensely powerful by age two. Cal's whole sense of security and trust has been thrown in disarray, and he can't manage what is about to take place. His emotions are overwhelming him, and he is clingy with his mother and withdraws into a five o'clock sleep. His cold shoulder to Daria, his trusted child-minder, suggests the anger that he feels at losing her. He can't possibly express this at his young age, so Cal's action—exhaustion—reveals the meaning behind his behavior.

Step five in Parental Intelligence is problem solving. Cal's well-being is at stake. His parents must face their essential task of creating yet another transition for his care. As a solution, Cal's mother researches childcare and finds two wonderful women who care for a small number of young children in one of their homes. Cal's mother not only stays with Cal at the new day care home for his first few days—so he can get acclimated—but she also decides to work from home two days a week. This allows her to spend more time with Cal on her own. As one of the partners in her business, Cal's mother can make an executive decision so that Cal only has to stay with the new caretakers three days a week. He does develop separation anxiety at first, crying sadly when his mother had to leave him for several weeks, but soon adjusted and found he could trust again. Cal even gave his mother the cold shoulder when she dropped him off at childcare—that same cold shoulder he had given to Daria when she was leaving. However, Cal's mother was wise and didn't pressure Cal, and he slowly adapted to his new environment and care.

(For a more detailed account of this story, read chapter five in *Unlocking Parental Intelligence: Finding Meaning in Your Child's Behavior*.)

LIDIA

At 7:00 a.m. Lidia's first alarm clock buzzes by her bed. She presses the snooze button, barely aware she's doing it. She has another alarm clock across the room, because she knows the one on her nightstand doesn't do the trick. In fact, getting up in the morning has become quite an event. Her mother admires that Lidia doesn't want to depend on her mother to wake her up, but inevitably she gets involved. Lidia paradoxically awakens exhausted! No matter how much sleep she can fit in, it isn't enough for the strenuous activities she's engaged in. She's certainly fit and eats well, but all her activities—except violin—weigh on her budding musculature. Each morning her mother must coax her to get dressed and eat a hearty breakfast. They don't argue, but they aren't exactly enjoying each other's company either.

Lidia is a spirited eight-year-old who does well in school and engages in many extracurricular activities: gymnastics, ballet, violin lessons, and lacrosse. This means five evenings a week and on Saturday mornings she is fully scheduled. Lidia loves all her activities and prides herself on her performance in all. She hopes to join the lacrosse travel team next year. Her mother not only feels the drudgery of chauffeuring or finding others to take her daughter to all these activities, but she observes that Lidia is usually exhausted and barely able to eat dinner and do homework before falling asleep, often at her desk. Lidia has begun to get minor illnesses too often, according to the pediatrician who brings this to Lidia's parents' attention.

Stepping back, step one of Parental Intelligence, Lidia's parents aren't really bewildered by her exhaustion, but they are concerned—especially when the pediatrician offers her worry to the equation. This pattern of scheduling has prevented Lidia from having play dates and generally hanging out. Lidia's parents find they barely have time to have conversations with Lidia except when driving in the car.

Self-reflecting, step two of Parental Intelligence, both parents realize they want to give their child all the advantages of learning various skills and having fun that their parents could not offer them when they were growing up. They have been determined since Lidia's toddlerhood to give Lidia every imaginable educational toy and preschool invention that could be found. By age three, Lidia was in full-time preschool and visited the library's events on the weekends. But at this point, Lidia's parents are finally beginning to question whether all of their scheduling is for Lidia or for themselves—to in some way make up for, through their daughter, what they feel they missed out on.

Understanding Lidia's mind, step three of Parental Intelligence, is difficult. Lidia claims she loves everything she does and is usually at the top of the groups in her performance, but she complains she doesn't really have friends to confide in. She isn't being invited to lots of birthday parties or sleepovers and feels left out. Her activities are in different towns than her school is—except for lacrosse, where some of her teammates are in her class.

Understanding her development, step four of Parental Intelligence, is also complex. At age eight she is straining a body that is still growing, and her pediatrician expresses concern that it may be too much. The doctor feels that all the physical exertion on Lidia's slim body may cause injuries that she is too young to endure. Lacrosse is particularly demanding, and if she gets on to the travel team then it will mean daily practices. Also considering a regular school day followed by gymnastics and ballet, her body is being pulled and stretched extensively.

Lidia's parents realize they have to problem solve, step five of Parental Intelligence, in order to protect their daughter from their scheduling of her life. Lidia is reluctant to have this talk, because she has absorbed her parents' wishes to never feel left out of every opportunity; Lidia has become a perfectionist. However, one quiet Sunday afternoon Lidia's parents decide to have a picnic lunch at a park nearby to spend some quality time together. As an only child, Lidia finds time with her parents special, because they work hard during the week. She is also quite exhausted by the time Sunday rolls around. So, they all sleep in and then have fun planning their lunchtime excursion. Once they are all in the car, Lidia's dad puts on some rock music, so different than the classical music Lidia is accustomed to at ballet. Lidia moves her body around in the car—despite her seat belt—and her father whistles along while her mother laughs and relaxes.

Once at the park, they lay out a big blanket and their hearty feast. First, they just talk about the park and plan on taking a bike ride later in the day. But finally, Dad has the courage to bring up the subject of over-scheduling. Lidia protests, "I like all that I do, and I do it really well. Why do you think we should change things? I promise I'll get up on my own from now on. I like to be independent and actually object when you [Mommy] try to help me get dressed."

Her mother replies, "I do understand that you like to be independent, and for eight years old, you really are! But tell us more truthfully what it's like for you when you try to wake up."

"I set two alarms as you know, but even though I try really hard to get out of bed, that second alarm just rings and rings. I can hardly move. Sometimes my calves ache from ballet, and my neck muscles even hurt from gymnastics. I hate to admit that I feel any of that. I want to be an Olympic star someday. Wouldn't that please you both?"

Dad says, "You've never told us these high aspirations. Olympic star! I can imagine it, but Olympic athletes usually focus on one sport, not several. Also, what's this about pleasing us?"

"I know you and Mommy take pleasure in all I do and constantly say 'just do your best,' but really I think that means 'be the best.' Don't you really mean that deep down?"

"NO!" both parents exclaim at once. Lidia's mother starts to cry and in between the tears says, "Lidia, I don't love you because of what you do or don't do. I love you always and forever—no matter what you choose. I think you mistook our enthusiasm for your activities for something more than we ever intended. You have our approval no matter how well you do at everything—including your schoolwork. Please don't think we are pressuring you to be perfect."

"I want to be perfect, and that's why I do my best. I think perfect is perfect! I know I need a lot of carbs to have the energy for my stuff, but sometimes I think I eat too much pasta and cheese and will get fat."

Her parents look at each other realizing an eating disorder could be in the making and that their over-scheduling is not the only problem. Lidia's perfectionistic standards are over-the-top, and they must address this problem seriously before it develops into something dire.

Dad adds, "I know sometimes you complain you don't get enough time just to hang out with girls, go to sleepovers, and stay up late for fun. What about all that?"

"I know I've said that, and I do mean it. I kind of feel left out in school when the kids fool around at recess. I sort of don't know how to fool around and just laugh and goof-off. It's like I never learned how to relax. Does this make any sense?"

As her daughter is talking, Lidia's mother feels proud that they all have a close enough relationship to be talking so openly. She's also glad no one has rushed in to try and solve particular problems yet, because so much is coming forth from Lidia. It is hard to define just yet what the priorities should be concerning her daughter's perfectionism, her wish for their approval, her wish to be an Olympic star, her wish for more friends, and her socializing self-doubts. *Thank goodness for Parental Intelligence or we would have rushed in and just changed her schedule without realizing the depths of her concerns.*

Instead of jumping in with his ideas, Dad wisely begins the problem-solving process by asking Lidia what she thinks can be done so she's a happier girl: "Lidia, you have told us so much today that we didn't know. I'm sorry you have kept so many worries to yourself. Where should we begin to help you feel better about yourself and feel less pressure to be perfect?"

"Oh, Daddy, I don't know. Maybe I should think hard if there's one sport that I really favor. I would like to have at least one or even two afternoons with nothing to do except play with other girls. Is that bad?"

"Oh my," says Dad. "Of course not. That's a great beginning to solving some of this. It's begun to sound more like stress than fun. Even your pediatrician is worried about you."

"Really? Why didn't you tell me? I think I get too many colds and sometimes want to just stay home in bed for the day, but I didn't realize that was realistic."

Lidia's mother joins in at this point. "It's very realistic. You are an exhausted child. We must face that together and monitor our expectations for you. I like the idea of focusing on one sport. Do you have a sense of what would be a possible choice?"

"Actually, I would really like to be on the travel team for lacrosse, because that's based on school friends who I could really get to know. I'd be at practice many days a week, and traveling to other states seems exciting. It would take a toll on you, too, though. You'd be travelling, too. Would you mind?"

"Sweetheart," her mother chimes in, "It would be a pleasure to take you and your friends to these trips. It *is* exciting. Could you put the idea of being an Olympiad on hold for a while and just enjoy what you do now rather than try to be the best? I know you'll succeed and we'll all get a charge out of that, but being part of a team is special, too."

Dad sums up a bit: "It's near the end of the school year, so let's not make changes now abruptly. We have the summer to think things over more. Would you like to go to a lacrosse camp and see if indeed you do like a few weeks of that? Then we can make more knowledgeable choices. Take a break from ballet and gymnastics for the summer if you agree. What about violin?"

"I like the idea of the four-week lacrosse camp. Can I go to one where you sleep over? Then I'll get to know the girls better. I can skip violin during that month of July, but I wouldn't want to give it up. In August I can resume the violin and then we'll decide what else to include. How does that sound?"

Both Lidia's parents were delighted with their plan. They were glad that they gave their daughter the chance to express her ideas before they chimed in. The plan had a tentativeness to it that would allow Lidia to experiment rather than make a certain decision. Also, they knew now that they had to make sure to speak to her differently, so she doesn't think approval is so high on their list. They never intended to have her worry about their approval; it was always such a given. Furthermore, they later discuss Lidia's diet plan with the pediatrician, so that Lidia steers away from an eating disorder, with that sense of perfectionism lingering on.

Problem solving the Parental Intelligence Way was certainly the right road for this family. They all shared honestly their worries and pleasures, and it is clear young Lidia is on her way to becoming a more relaxed, less exhausted child.

LAURA

Laura is a lanky, eleven-year-old girl, taller than many girls and boys her age at five foot four. She is entering middle school and doesn't feel like she knows who she is anymore. She's scared to meet all the new kids from the other elementary schools, mainly because her body seems to be changing so fast. She wonders every morning how she'll look and feel. On top of that, she feels exhausted most of the time, even though she generally gets eight hours of sleep each night.

What Laura and her parents don't know is that by puberty, nine and a half hours of sleep are necessary—with some kids needing twelve or thirteen hours a night. Laura's parents have four children all older than Laura, so you'd think they would know this, but they just weren't thinking about Laura in particular.

Laura's body is changing so rapidly. When Laura looks in the mirror she thinks, *My hips are getting wide. Am I fat? Why am I taller than everyone? Also, I'm perspiring and getting some hair under my arms. It's embarrassing. I don't want anyone to know. I hope Mommy thinks that she just misplaced the deodorant I stole from her bathroom. I definitely don't want to talk about that, but we have to go clothes shopping. My jeans are too tight and short. Ugh. Who am I anyway?*

Labor Day is only a week away and Laura tells her mother, "I don't want to start sixth grade. The work is going to be too hard, I can't imagine having lots of teachers, I won't know most of the girls, I'm kind of afraid of boys, and I feel so ugly!" She has to force this last part out of her mouth. Laura's mother had been thinking mostly about her own work schedule that would conflict with Laura's school day. Plus, she had her four other kids who were teenagers to think about, ages thirteen, fifteen, seventeen, and eighteen.

The eighteen-year-old is starting college, and that is the biggest shift in the family that everyone will have to get used to, thought Laura's mother. But when Laura spoke up, her mother stepped back and thought, *Oh my. Is she my forgotten sweet girl? She has been rather quiet all summer, spending time babysitting for a neighbor and being proud of making money on a regular basis. I haven't given enough thought to how her body is changing. I imagine she'll get her period soon. Also, her oldest sibling is the one she confides in, my only other daughter, and she'll be away at school shortly. She definitely doesn't confide in her three brothers. In fact, she does her best to ignore them. I have noticed that she always seems exhausted even though she seems to sleep well, and she isn't really working out or doing anything particularly strenuous. What is going on with her?*

Laura's mother shares with her husband in confidence what Laura had said, telling him not to bring it up; this was girl talk. Self-reflecting, he says, "We're missing something here. When our older daughter reached this stage, we were much more focused on her. She was the first, and all the bodily changes were so new to us. We must get back in the game. Laura is going through puberty! I'm sorry, dear, but this is your province—though I'm here to support you. I guess my job is to reassure her that she looks pretty without sounding too obvious about it. I know our minds are on college shopping, but definitely take Laura to the stores right away before school starts."

Laura's mother is so glad to talk to her husband. Self-reflecting reminds her that she, too, was the youngest of five kids and felt forgotten during her pubescent years. She only had older brothers, which had been such a pain because she was sure no one noticed or cared about her. She must have wanted to forget about that difficult time and so was blind to what was happening to Laura. But, no more short-sightedness. Laura needed her now!

Laura was greatly relieved when her mother told her that Saturday was "just for them." Everyone else would have to rely on Dad and fend for themselves. They would go out for a sushi lunch—Laura's favorite—chat, and then shop all afternoon.

Saturday morning comes, and exhausted Laura is anxious to go out with her mother. Laura encourages her mother to leave by eleven for an early lunch, because she doesn't even know which stores to go to with her cock-eyed body image. At lunch, Laura confesses she doesn't want to eat too much, even her favorite sashimi-sushi platter, because she is afraid she is getting fat. "Mommy, I think my hips are too big. I look down at them all day. I'm not as skinny as I usually think of myself. Maybe I should get T-shirts that hide my belly."

Laura's mother responds, "Laura, you're growing into the shape of a young woman, not getting fat. We all have hips and curves. You're just not used to it. We will adjust your size and you'll feel better. You don't have to hide your changing body under big shirts. I know you don't feel it, but you look very pretty and can wear all kinds of 'in' clothes—even tight-ish ones that you see on the mannequins in the store windows."

"I'd really like that," Laura says blushing, "Oh, how do I say this? Am I getting *sexy*?" she whispers. Her mother tries not to laugh because that would shut Laura down. Instead she says as seriously as she can muster, "Yes. You have a lovely figure. You're just not used to it, because you changed so much and so quickly. But that's what happens to a lot of girls your age. You feel alone, but you're not. Let's go to the chic stores in that little mall downtown." Laura brightens up, feeling her mother really understands, and finishes eating quickly, excited to get out there to those shops. Laura's mother has a lot of experience dressing her older daughter and feels she can understand her youngest easily. Laura's mind was an open book!

To Laura's surprise, Laura's mother takes her first to the lingerie department to have her fitted properly for new bras. The sales woman is so expert at working with young girls that Laura loses her embarrassment and begins to feel some confidence. Now her shirts will look nice! Then they go to the junior department and try on a lot of different jeans and shirts—and even some skirts and blouses that Laura never would have thought to try. She notices other girls in the store wearing these outfits and is pleased that her mother is so self-assured and didn't hesitate to pick out a variety of styles.

After their successful excursion, Laura's dad compliments his wife on their young daughter's high spirits. However, he is concerned about the exhaustion that Laura shows once again. He can't attribute that to shopping. Laura's parents realize now that they still aren't focusing enough on Laura's physical development, and they check on sleeping patterns for girls going through puberty. Laura's parents google information about sleep at puberty, and together, eyes on the screen, they are shocked to see that the seven or eight hours Laura is getting aren't nearly enough. Laura very willingly goes to sleep earlier so that she can get up for her babysitting feeling wide awake. This was an easy one to solve once Laura and her parents attended to her stage of development.

Laura's problems seemed to be solved with the choice of the shopping excursion, but it was really much more than that. Shopping involved giving Laura a chance to express her confusion about her changing body, understand her exhaustion, and relieve the embarrassment she felt about her awkwardness. Both parents recognized these feelings, and her father supported her mother emotionally as she took on the task of understanding Laura's mind. When Laura felt understood, she felt better. She learned she wasn't alone but that most girls her age were going through the same confusions. She also felt better finding out that awkward could mean sexy—a revelation for an eleven-year-old!

We have seen that exhaustion is a symptom of varied problems with a wide range of meanings. Exhausted Cal did not need more sleep. He needed attention to his feelings of loss that overwhelmed him at his young age. Exhausted Lidia couldn't get enough sleep because her schedule was too full—which was the result of her wishes for perfectionism and parental approval. Exhausted Laura did need more sleep to halt her exhaustion, but the meanings behind her journey through puberty focused on her self-image. Using the Parental Intelligence Way to examine your child's exhaustion reveals the underlying meanings behind the exhaustion, a behavior we are becoming more aware of and that is prevalent through childhood. As we turn to adolescence once again, we will dive more into exhaustion and its many underlying meanings.

CHAPTER THREE

LEARNING ABOUT THE EXHAUSTED ADOLESCENT THE PARENTAL INTELLIGENCE WAY

LESLIE

Fourteen-year-old Leslie drags herself up the stairs to land on her bed right after school on most days, falling into a deep sleep that can last for three hours. She's always shocked that it's six o'clock when she opens her drowsy eyes and that her mother is calling her down to dinner. Like most good academic kids, she can't sleep like this every day, because she is a member of the debate team and editor of the school paper. She almost always feels exhausted. Sometimes she falls asleep in class, only to get kicked under her desk by her friend to wake her up. At night she sleeps like a rock. Her mother thinks her problem is that she's picking the wrong friends who aren't as smart and goal oriented as she is. She fears her daughter is getting lazy. But her mother is off the mark this time.

Leslie and her mother have constant arguments about these friends. Her mother is afraid she's learning bad habits and is going to get into trouble sexually if she doesn't regroup with her old steady friends, who are polite and steadfast with their schoolwork. But Leslie needs to experiment with different kids. She feels it's really harmless, but she and her mother of course disagree.

Leslie spends hours a day preoccupied with her anxieties: she worries about expiration dates on foods, avoiding any leftovers, and separates each food from the others on her plate. She also spends a lot of time lining up her old stuffed animals in a specific order on her shelf. She's begun skipping lunch at school entirely, because she likes eating by herself to avoid inquiries from her friends about these habits. But they all actually accept her compulsions and treat her normally. Her mother doesn't realize that she's adding to Leslie's obsessive thoughts by constantly telling Leslie to wash her hands after school and to avoid those nasty germs all around her that will get her sick. Leslie has now added this obsession to her repertoire and uses her shirt to open doors; she doesn't want to touch the doorknobs in school that everyone is handling. She's become what kids call a germaphobe.

Leslie is well liked and no one except her therapist knows about the excessive sleep. Her exhaustion is hidden, because her mother thinks she is doing homework and visiting kids on the computer. But her mother is still worried about her. Leslie's excessive sleep interferes with her homework, which causes its own problems because Leslie is a good student with a lot of advanced placement classes. If Leslie doesn't write something perfectly, according to her excessive standards, she rips up her work and rewrites it. Writing on the computer helps her, but then she gets preoccupied with the margins, spacing, and spellcheck—once again deleting all her work until it's perfect. On the standardized tests that have become so common, she must pencil in the little answer circles perfectly or she erases her work and does it over. This takes time from solving the problems that she's supposed to be focusing on.

What does exhaustion have to do with OCD (obsessive-compulsive disorder)? Well, Leslie is avoiding her obsessive thoughts and compulsions just to get a mental break from them. Sleep is her escape.

Leslie's mother is a dedicated parent. She stays at home while her husband works long hours. She desperately thinks that the problem is Leslie's friend group, and she likes Leslie's therapist but thinks the therapist is not worried enough about Leslie's peer life. Leslie's mother doesn't realize it's Leslie's OCD that's leading to Leslie's exhaustion and severe anxiety.

After a full year of the therapist's interventions, both parents are called in once again, only now for more frequent parent sessions. The therapist is firm and caring about Leslie and wants her parents to face the fact that Leslie's OCD is real, is distressing Leslie all the time, and is interfering with her daily life—even the academics that her parents prize. Leslie openly shares with her parents all her inner pressures, no longer caring about their approval. She needs more help, and medication is clearly warranted.

Stepping back hadn't helped Leslie's parents, because they reinforced what they thought was her real problem: friend choices. They missed the exhaustion, and Leslie hid her scrupulous obsessive habits. Finally, when Leslie's misery was too much for her to bear and Leslie pointed out a list of her compulsions, her parents stepped back and saw the patterns they'd been dismissing. Self-reflecting, they realized that they didn't want to see their daughter as "having a mental illness," like their own parents had. They didn't want to believe their own child suffered with those same characteristics. But once Leslie and her therapist helped Leslie's parents to understand Leslie's irrational mind-set, her parents cried and came around to giving Leslie all the help she needed.

Leslie's parents discussed Leslie's stage of development with her pediatrician, who wisely advised them that her experimenting with different circles of friends was normal, but her OCD was not, and it was deeply distressing their daughter. Problem solving effectively, with the therapist's help, Leslie's parents had Leslie consult with a psychopharmacologist. Leslie was prescribed Paxil, a selective serotonin reuptake inhibitor (SSRI) that fortunately worked quickly and effectively for Leslie. However, quickly is relative, because it takes time to slowly move to a high enough dosage that is effective; however, by the following year, Leslie was nearly symptom-free, was thriving academically, and had a mixed group of friends, and her exhaustion had slowly vanished. Thus, through effective problem solving, the parents were able to help their daughter combine the therapy she needed (such as Cognitive Behavioral Therapy) with medication to alter the over-arching problem of OCD that led her to use sleep as a psychological escape (which looked like exhaustion).

This troubling situation points to the importance of step two, self-reflecting, in the Parental Intelligence tool kit. Because the parents had both lived through at least one of their parents having OCD symptoms, they desperately didn't want to face that their own child could be genetically predisposed to the same problems. With the therapist's parental guidance over an extended period, Leslie's folks faced their own distress at seeing a multigenerational mental disorder.

This process was painful for both Leslie and her parents, but with enough time, dedicated therapeutic intervention, and Parental Intelligence, they became more open-minded. They could take a good look at their own inner selves as well as their child's inner world. Leslie was fortunate that the SSRI did not have any side effects for her and that her first trial at medication was successful. It's important to know that often several different

SSRIs have to be tried before the right choice and dosage is found.

Leslie's exhaustion was a key element because it pointed to deeper difficulties. Teenagers do need a lot more sleep than most parents are aware of, which we will soon discover was Wade's plight, but for Leslie it was just a symptom of a more serious problem.

WADE

As a sixteen-year-old superathlete, Wade was a very popular kid. His basketball talents were prestigious in his state. He was headed for a career in basketball by all the recruiters' measures, even at sixteen. But despite his many coaches' good advice, he never had enough sleep. He was an exhausted superstar.

His parents didn't want to thwart his career goals, and indeed were pleased with their athletic prodigy, but they found his exhaustion disconcerting. On top of that, his grades were dropping, which could interfere with the expected basketball scholarship he needed for college. Stepping back, they believed he was just working out too hard and that all his practices after school and on weekends were beyond reasonable. They were fully self-reflective and did not want their hopes for their son's success to lead him to overdo what his body was capable of. It was studying and understanding his stage of development that brought light to the subject of his exhaustion.

Siri Carpenter (American Psychological Association, *Monitor* Staff, October 2001, 42) reported the following about teenagers' sleep:

> For most, the alarm clock buzzes by 6:30 a.m., a scant seven hours after they went to bed. Many students board the school bus before 7 a.m. and are in class by 7:30.
>
> In adults, such meager sleep allowances are known to affect day-to-day functioning in myriad ways. In adolescents, who are biologically driven to sleep longer and later than adults do, the effects of insufficient sleep are likely to be even more dramatic—so much so that some sleep experts contend that the nation's early high school start times, increasingly common, are tantamount to abuse.

"Almost all teenagers, as they reach puberty, become walking zombies because they are getting far too little sleep," comments Cornell University psychologist James B. Maas, one of the nation's leading sleep experts. "There can be little question that sleep deprivation has negative effects on adolescents. . . . Insufficient sleep has also been shown to cause difficulties in school, including disciplinary problems, sleepiness in class, and poor concentration. What good does it do to try to educate teenagers so early in the morning?" asks Maas. "You can be giving the most stimulating, interesting lectures to sleep-deprived kids early in the morning or right after lunch, when they're at their sleepiest, and the overwhelming drive to sleep replaces any chance of alertness, cognition, memory, or understanding."

Recent research has also revealed an association between sleep deprivation and poorer grades. In a 1998 survey of more than 3,000 high school students, for example, psychologist A.R. Wolfson, of the College of the Holy Cross, and M.A. Carskadon, of Brown University Medical School, found that students who reported that they were getting Cs, Ds and Fs in school obtained about twenty-five minutes less sleep and went to bed about forty minutes later than students who reported they were getting As and Bs.

Given this information (that will be more detailed in chapter eight), it became clear to Wade, his parents, and even his coaches that he was sleep-deprived. He needed at least ten hours of sleep each night, given his age and his extensive work-outs, in order to meet the growing demands of his body. Because of his academic workload and athletic practices, Wade was getting more like seven hours each night—which was not giving his muscles time to rebuild, even with his unusual body type. He was veritably playing basketball exhausted!

Once this information was understood, problem solving was easy. His parents stopped waking him up early on weekends because they felt he should be productive, and Wade tried to make up for some of the weekday sleep he couldn't fit in. But this isn't the only tack to take; the coaches had to monitor his physical workload so that he could get home in time to eat a very nutritious dinner, do his homework, and get the ten hours of sleep he needed. There was even the beginning of a reevaluation of the school day hours for teenagers in that area due to Wade's experience and the similar experiences of other kids his age. Many parents spoke up about it at the school's parent-teacher meetings, greatly affecting the powers that be in the district. The superintendent, especially, took the lead in spearheading a movement to reexamine the school schedule for adolescents in his district.

LEE

Lee is a seventeen-year-old high school senior at the top of his class. He will probably be valedictorian. But his soaring academic record doesn't give him the certainty he wants that he'll get into a top Ivy League university.

He lives in a very competitive region of the United States where hundreds of kids in his geographic area also have super-high grades, perfect SAT scores, and a multitude of accomplishments outside the school curriculum. These students are overly preoccupied with their standing in the whole state, not just their school. Top universities want diversity, and Lee knows that his résumé—while outstanding—is still not ensuring acceptance. So, he applied to seventeen schools!

Seventeen applications, tutoring for SATs, five advanced-placement classes, and language proficiency in three languages all took a great deal of time. He is getting about six hours of sleep each night, hardly enough for this level of activity. Furthermore, he works after school at a science lab, which makes him stand out even further among his peers, where he won a science competition that ranked him in the top 2 percent of the nation's science competitors. Lee is a high-powered, ambitious teenager who is exhausted!

Not surprisingly his parents are both ambitious, hard-working adults who have always had very high expectations for their brilliant son. They indeed pushed him very hard from elementary school onwards, living beyond their means so that Lee could go to a very special school for gifted kids. They had not gone to private schools themselves but did believe that college competition was greater for their son than it had been for them. They are determined that Lee should be a rich, successful adult in his twenties and thirties.

Lee emulated his parent's high standards, cared deeply for their approval, and sacrificed much of his social life to meet their goals for him. Unfortunately, such pressures took their toll and Lee is not happy. He is persistently worn out, has many headaches, and worries incessantly that he will disappoint his parents and therefore himself. He barely has time for socializing, resulting in an awkwardness that left him with few friends. In fact, he has acquaintances, not really close friendships, and suffers with low self-esteem and social anxiety. His exhaustion is increased due to his social tension, because he has trouble falling asleep when he worries that he wasn't liked. During middle school he was bullied severely as a "weird nerd" and even got closed in a locker by some terribly mean boys for what seemed like an endless amount of time. This experience traumatized him, adding some claustrophobia to his social anxiety.

Lee's parents did comfort him after the bullying experiences, but they didn't let down on their high academic expectations because of the rewards they expected for him in the long run. They both grew up in lower-middle-class homes where money was always an issue. They did not want this to be their son's life, but they missed out on looking at his general well-being and dismissed his angst.

One Saturday morning, Lee slept through his first Ivy League interview—to his amazement—and his parents awakened him at noon. He was beside himself crying, and he called appropriately to apologize and reschedule. But his parents were furious. They weren't accustomed to Lee needing them to wake him up for anything. This was an aberration from his usual dutiful life. He tried to seek their comfort, saying he had hardly slept through the night because he was so worried about this first interview. He also pointed out that he had awaken with a start when they stirred him. Plus, he had a pounding headache.

Although mindful of Parental Intelligence, Lee's parents usually passed the five steps off as too coddling for their superior son. But they were indeed shaken when they saw Lee sobbing after they finished yelling at him.

"Lee," his father said rather harshly, "Stop acting like a baby and get yourself together. You're seventeen years old and headed for a great life. What is there to cry about? A missed appointment? The gentleman said it was fine to reschedule, no harm is done."

Lee replied while still crying, "Dad, I don't think you know me as well as you think you do. I'm an idiot. I can't get along with other kids, they think I'm arrogant when I'm actually shy. And even if I do get into your super Ivy League school, I probably won't have any friends!"

Lee's mother had never seen her son in such a state or so forthright with her husband—who was quite domineering, even with her. While her husband and son were arguing, she thought, *Maybe Parental Intelligence isn't so foolhardy. Stepping back, I can't forget his bullying experiences in middle school, and he never smiles now that I think about it. The pressure has gotten to him. He's one miserable, brilliant, but exhausted child. If we don't listen carefully to him, he could get into a great school, only to have a nervous breakdown! He's trembling. Does my husband even notice that?*

Lee's mother put her arm on her husband's back and gently suggested they leave Lee alone for a while to rest and compose himself. She didn't really want to leave her son alone, but she had to remove her husband so he could collect himself and become self-reflective. Lee looked into his mother's eyes, felt her compassion, realized her motivation, and was relieved to be by himself for a while. In fact, he fell back to sleep for two hours.

Lee's mother was as ambitious for Lee as her husband, but she had a softer side, too. She made her spouse and herself some tea and sandwiches and said they needed to have a serious talk. She spoke about how her father was a tough construction worker who did the best for her family, and she knew her husband wanted much more for her son. But she said, "We have to look at the costs now before Lee goes away to school and is on his own with less emotional support. We must face that he doesn't have friends. We are his major allies but aren't acting that way. Social life is just as important as academic life, and Lee isn't even dating at all. He's going to university without a social backbone. He's in for a very lonely experience."

To her amazement, Lee's father teared up. "I'm so incompetent as a father. I try hard, but it's a miserable way I treat Lee. I try and build him up but am always dismissing my thoughts about how awkward he feels— even to me—when we are talking with other people. He's polite and quiet. Too quiet. It's as if he doesn't know how to converse amiably with people. This is kind of a light bulb for me, but maybe he's afraid to be inter- viewed and so slept through it. His lack of social confi- dence may become apparent in an interview. I wonder how that might negate all his academic prowess."

Lee's mother spoke up, clearly focused now on what was needed. They had to understand their dear son's mind and respond carefully and lovingly. "Let's wait until dinner and then have a talk with Lee and express our apologies for pushing him so hard. Let's invite him to tell us what he's been worrying about. Remember not to interrupt him or criticize him. We must hear him out and then support his wishes. We know what our dreams are for him, but what are *his* aspirations and dreams? Let's become good listeners. We're not so great at that, you know."

At dinner, Dad began, "Lee, we're sorry you're having such a difficult emotional time. I admit I don't pay too much attention to feelings. I try to hide my own, and I'm afraid I've dismissed yours. Tell us as openly as you can what's really worrying you. I promise we won't interrupt or blame you for anything you say."

Lee replied honestly, the only way he knew how. "I'm very lonely. I keep up with all the work but always feel down. The other kids ignore me; no one bullies me anymore, but I'm a loner. You don't know how solitary I've become."

Lee's mother spoke up quietly and sensitively, "Tell us more about what your days are like. We want to help you feel better and not get those headaches and get more sleep."

"I don't know what to say. I can't change my path now and don't want to. I do want to be a big success in life, but I need to learn how to talk with people. Interviewers might find me really boring and certainly not witty and engaging. What if they care about that?

Even if they don't, I do. I want to enjoy college. When we see where I get accepted and I am confident I will get into some good schools, let's visit them while the classes are in session and get a feel for the kind of life I'll be living. I don't even know if I want a country or city school. I don't know myself very well. I have a lot of knowledge and I'm proficient in so many areas of learning, but I don't know how to get along with people. Maybe I need a small school to feel comfortable in. I can't imagine a huge university. I'll be lost."

Understanding Lee's mind like this was a new experience for all of them. His parents realized that Lee's social development was like a younger child and that this was the problem. His exhaustion pointed to the kind of academic and work life he was living as well as his emotional life that they had dismissed.

Problem solving wasn't easy, but his parents tried. Dad said, "I agree we will visit as may schools as you want and find the right place for you to feel comfortable in. Small colleges can be just as prestigious as large universities. In fact, you might get a better education because more professors will be teaching the classes rather than large lectures by grad school assistant instructors. We have a lot of time to think about this all year, so let's all lighten up and remember we're in this together. I'm sorry, son, I've been such a curmudgeon.

Your mother is the warmer one, and we have to take her lead."

This was just the first of many conversations that the family had throughout the year. Lee's mother helped with some applications to ease his load, and they spent more time together doing things that were pleasurable—like they might do with a younger son. They went to the movies and out to dinner, and they encouraged him to join a fun club or two to meet other teenagers, not achieve anything in particular. With his parents' support, Lee slept better and ventured to have some conversations with other quieter kids at school, regardless of how brilliant or accomplished they were.

Lee's first year away from home would be hard for him. But he seemed to grow up a lot his senior year after his parents came out of their steadfast expectations for him. He made a few friends and even had fun at some graduation parties. He was accepted into nearly every school he applied to, and in the end he did choose Harvard. However, he focused on joining some small extracurricular activities where he could meet friends easily. He also carefully chose a low-key roommate by chatting on Facebook. The whole family mellowed, and Lee kept close contact with his parents during his freshman year so that he could continue to feel supported emotionally.

Three exhausted teens. All with different temperaments, goals, and parent expectations. Common to all these busy parents was their initial reluctance to jump on the bandwagon of Parental Intelligence because of their own needs to shield themselves from their inner motivations. However, the five steps of Parental Intelligence helped each teen and his or her parents find their way through the journey of adolescence quite successfully once they undertook the significance of their parenting styles. Helping teens find their own way when parents have high hopes for them is a heartwarming, yet sometimes painful, path.

CHAPTER FOUR

EXHAUSTION AND CHILD AND ADOLESCENT DEVELOPMENT

Exhaustion is defined as extreme mental or physical fatigue. In *Pediatrics* (2012) from the American Academy of Pediatrics, it was found that kids today are not getting an adequate amount of sleep as a result of modern life and due to current technologies. No matter how much sleep children are getting, it is always assumed that they need more. Generally, the literature seems to agree on the following sleep needs:

Age	Recommended	May be appropriate
Preschoolers *3–5 years*	10 to 13 hours	8 to 9 hours; 14 hours
School-aged Children *6–13 years*	9 to 11 hours	7 to 8 hours; 12 hours
Teenagers *14–17 years*	8 to 10 hours	7 to 11 hours
Young Adults *18–25 years*	7 to 9 hours	6 to 11 hours

Babies, children, and adolescents need significantly more sleep than adults do in order to support their rapid mental and physical development. However, children often act as if they're not tired, resisting bedtime and becoming hyper as the evening goes on. All this can happen because the child *is* overtired. Some kids do indeed say they are tired or fall asleep on a couch or in a restaurant, but many often resist when parents say it's time for bed—especially if they are enjoying themselves. Instead of understanding their exhaustion, they become irritable and hyperactive because they don't know what is happening to their bodies. It's clearly the province of their parents to explain that they are indeed tired and need their rest so that they can be alert and energetic the next day. Such explanations are often not given, and parents respond with yelling and threats of punishment. Following the guidelines of Parental Intelligence, parents might successfully step back and recognize that their frequent bedtime arguments may mean that their child perceives bedtime as punitive instead of a necessary physical routine. Understanding your child's mind-set about bedtime is helpful, because if you hear why your child thinks she has a bedtime, you can straighten out any misperceptions of your rules that pertain to essential rest needs. When children know *why* they must sleep, they are much more inclined to listen than if they are forced to adhere to, what for them are, inexplicable parental dictates.

Sleep times should never be viewed as punishments by our children, because that would skew a realistic understanding of a body's need for rest. Instead, it can't be emphasized enough how helpful it is for busy parents to discuss the reasons for sleep and come to reasonable agreements about bedtimes. Bedtime routines help inordinately in securing children's needs for security and emotional regulation when it is time for sleep. Reading to children after finishing their hygiene tasks is most common and helpful. It is also known that reading to children—even when they can read for themselves—not only settles them down and induces restfulness, but also results in kids who want to read—a measure of intelligence.

In *Paediatrics & Child Health* (2008), Dr. Sheri M. Findley reviews the complaint of overtiredness in teens. She reports that ". . . sleepiness is defined as 'an increased tendency to fall asleep' and is generally considered the opposite of alertness. Subjectively, the rates of daytime sleepiness among teens vary between 10 percent and 40 percent, tending to increase from early to later adolescence. Objectively, sleepiness is measured using the multiple sleep latency test, in which the patient attempts to nap under fixed ideal conditions, and sleep latency (time to the onset of sleep) is measured." Supported by anecdotes told by teens, objective measures using the multiple sleep latency test confirm that many teens do, in fact, have a higher than expected (and unhealthy) tendency to fall asleep during the day. Not surprisingly, the usual cause of excess sleepiness is insufficient or inadequate sleep—both very common during the teen years. A recent publication of the American Academy of Pediatrics' Working Group on Sleepiness in Adolescents/Young Adults summarized that

> teens need nine hours to ten hours of sleep per night for optimal functioning, but for a variety of reasons, many do not get this. Lifestyle factors contributing to this problem include early start times for most high schools and

an increasing amount of extracurricular and employment demands on many adolescents. The availability of highly entertaining computer and video games as well as late night socializing via the Internet also contribute to the unwillingness to get to bed at a decent time to get the recommended nine hours to ten hours of sleep. Such teens may find napping in the afternoon unavoidable, giving them an untimely sense of energy late in the day, further contributing to the late nights. Teenagers with insufficient sleep typically catch up on sleep on weekends, with very late rise times on weekend mornings.

Late rising times on weekends is often an unnecessary source of arguments between teens and parents. When parents understand this is needed, not a measure of laziness or unproductivity, then their teenagers can feel understood and get the sleep they need. Additionally, parents have one less power skirmish to handle. Discuss with your teen that you understand their late morning—or even early afternoon—sleep in during the weekend is because they aren't getting what they need during the weekdays. Again looking to Parental Intelligence, a teen's excessive weekend sleep shouldn't be a source of arguments and parent-teen clashes, but a time when adolescents can feel that their parents understand them and their various activities, responsibilities, and school loads.

In 2000, the National Sleep Foundation summarized important sleep information for parents of teens:

1. Adolescents require at least as much sleep as they did as preadolescents (in general, 8.5 to 9.25 hours each night).

2. Daytime sleepiness increases even when an adolescent's schedule provides for optimal amounts of sleep.

3. Adolescents' sleep patterns reveal a phase delay—that is, a tendency toward later times, for both sleeping and waking. Studies show that the typical high school student's natural time to fall asleep is 11:00 p.m. or later. This often results in many parent-teen arguments, because parents are not aware of this fact.

This phase delay is a source of controversy in many school districts where the teenagers start school earlier than the younger children due to sports and after school activities that require later school days for the teens. While this may be the case, this is not in keeping with their natural sleep cycle and may result in sleepiness during the school day, reducing cognitive function and concentration.

Children and adolescents acquire language, social, and motor skills at a rapid pace throughout their growing years. It can't be overemphasized that while adults need seven to nine hours of sleep per night, one-year-olds need about eleven to fourteen hours, preschoolers between ten and thirteen, school-age kids between nine and eleven, and teens between eight and ten. During these critical growth and learning periods, younger kids need a heavier dose of sleep for optimal development and alertness. A child or teen can't easily accumulate sleep deprivation and then log more hours of sleep later to make up for their sleep debt—though it's a good idea if you're sleep deprived. The best sleep habits are consistent, healthy routines to meet sleep needs nightly in order to stay on top of life's challenges daily.

EXHAUSTED KIDS OF PARENTS WITH MARITAL PROBLEMS

When parents are experiencing marital problems it often results in exhaustion for both children and parents. Children who are listening to parents argue at night often suffer from increased anxiety and, potentially, decreased sleep. Even if the fighting occurs when kids are sleeping, children awaken to the tense sounds of their parents' voices and imagine the worst. Some kids get out of bed to see what's going on when their parents aren't even aware of it. A child or teen peeking into their parents' bedroom to see their parents verbally attacking each other can be traumatic. Some kids yell and scream, "Stop it!" but most sneak back to bed undiscovered and have great difficulty falling back to sleep due to their worries, fears, and insecurities. Parents are often more powerful figures in their kids' lives than they ever imagine. At every developmental age, to see your parents out of control is frightening. Younger children don't have the cognitive capacity of adolescents to make sense of the turmoil. Additionally, the next morning when the children are overtired and arguments ensue between parents and kids about getting up, the parents often have no idea that it was *their* turmoil that caused the sleeplessness in their children.

Other parents enduring marital stress use the silent treatment, not talking to each other for days. Their children and teens clearly observe this behavior and often adopt it, causing increased tension in the household. This can, too, result in sleep restlessness and insufficient hours of rest. Healthy, normal development is impacted by the upsurge in exhaustion that results from family stress.

Parents with marital problems need to realize the impact their relationship has on their children. It may be necessary to seek help in individual and/or marital psychotherapy to relieve and work out their stress. Parents should be encouraged to have one-on-one conversations with their children and teens to learn about the worries and insecurities that may be resulting from their marital tension. In this instance especially, the third step in Parental Intelligence (understanding your child's mind) and the fourth step (understanding your child's development) aren't options. They are necessities. Honestly admitting to your children that "Mommy and Daddy aren't getting along but it's not your fault" is crucial. Your children may be unsettled and scared about facing the fact that their parents are at odds with each other, but this is better than shutting down communication between adults and kids—as if that keeps the marital tension hidden. Busy parents need to listen carefully to their kids' fears, which often concern whether their parents will get divorced. The question, "Who will take care of me?" from frightened children is inevitable. Luckily, even if divorce and custody battles are in their future, children will at least know that they can continue to ask questions and that they will be taken care of.

In the case of joint custody, children generally live in two households, another situation that often leads to exhaustion. Imagine this common scenario: The children spend a few days in the household of their parent who rises very early to get to work. Because of this early work schedule, this parent has to drop his kids off at his ex-spouse's home early in the morning, where they can stay until she goes to work. Then the children go to school, have extracurricular activities, and go to after-school care until the parent in charge that day comes home from work. These children have a long, long day without rest, only to get home for a quick dinner and homework before bed. It is unlikely that these children will get enough sleep. The results are:

- exhaustion
- sleep deprivation
- acting out, often in school
- decreased concentration
- disorganization of schoolwork
- a drop in grades

The only way to forestall these results is to build stringent rules into the divorce contract that define the sleep needs of each child. However, this is rarely done, because the divorced couple are focusing on their financial needs, dividing assets, the geography of their now divided homes, and their visitation rights. These tired children often end up feeling like baggage, dropped off from home to home to non-speaking adults who are supposed to make them feel secure.

Custody arrangements must be in the best interests of the children in order to work reasonably well. Depending on the hostilities that remain between the ex-spouses, this is or isn't feasible. Clearly psychotherapeutic help is warranted and needs to be maintained for the duration of the first year of divorce—at a minimum. Exhaustion is compounded by feelings of loss, a sense of helplessness or trauma, and the rapid rise of insecurity. Co-parenting where both parents use Parental Intelligence is ideal and can be achieved with divorced parents—whether they are in agreement about the end of their marriage or are more hostile. All divorced parents should seek therapeutic parental guidance on a regular, consistent basis and each member of their family should have a chance to speak at least weekly with the therapist(s). If possible, these therapy sessions would include both individual and family sessions. Divorce agreements should specify what kind of therapeutic help is required—and how much—so it is not left to chance.

EXHAUSTED KIDS IN DUAL-WORKING HOUSEHOLDS

When both parents work, which is most common today, schedules get very difficult. As in most developing families, each child is at a different level and requires a different amount of sleep. Plus, parents need sleep too. When parents forget to step back and view their kids' behaviors in the context of having two working parents with tight, rushed schedules, arguments about bedtimes increase and needless punishments ensue. To add to the stress, it often happens that no one in a dual working household seems to have downtime for some daily conversation and dialogue about each other's pleasures or fears. Luckily, some jobs relieve the tension with days for working at home and paid or unpaid maternity and paternity leave. And while household help with the physical care of the home, carefully planned childcare arrangements, and organized routines for taking kids to activities can surely help to manage the chaos, they can all be costly. Forgotten once again in this mix is each family member's need for enough sleep. If parents aren't careful, sleep and dialogue often become last on the to-do list, making exhaustion and rushing each other through the day par for the course.

If you find that these scenarios are common in your home, reread the first section of this chapter on the amount of sleep required for each developmental stage, review the principles of Parental Intelligence, and clearly factor in parent exhaustion. While this book focuses on our children, adults without enough sleep can hardly muster up the energy for parent-child relationships that need to be the first, not last, priority. The exhaustion examples in chapters two and three are reminders that situations needn't be dire if Parental Intelligence is uppermost on your minds. Using Parental Intelligence can help you keep in perspective that schedules will get thrown off for various unpredictable contingencies, kids will get sick, and parents will lose promotions, but with open dialogue, empathy for our children's needs remains intact.

CHAPTER FIVE

THE OVERSCHEDULED CHILD AND AN EMPHASIS ON SMART KIDS

*F*eeling emotionally secure and not overtired are important components of happiness that are often not considered when parents schedule their children's daily lives. It is important for busy parents, children, and teens to examine their goals when scheduling activities before and after school, as well as on weekends. As you schedule your daily lives, it is essential to look at your intentions as a parent, your child's intentions, and how your resulting plans will impact everyone psychologically. Changing external conditions, such as revising the schedule, might seem to work at first and must be considered, but if a family member cannot control or regulate her emotions well then fears and anxieties may return—despite the schedule change.

Let's think about the current situation in many geographic areas of the United States, where children are overscheduled, overwhelmed, at odds with their parents, and exhausted. The most important concerns parents should have are how their kids feel about themselves and the quality of their experiences. Pleasure is a feeling of contentment that children only achieve whenever expectations—physical and emotional—are met. However, this contentment is hard to reach through exhaustion. Examining the intentions and goals of both parents and their children is necessary when planning your daily schedules in order to avoid this exhaustion.

Let's take a step back and contemplate alternatives for an overscheduled child. Perhaps, for example, we might consider the child who has enough time to daydream—quite the opposite of a perpetually scheduled lifestyle. Psychologist Mihaly Csikszentmihalyi in his book *Flow* (1990) explains that daydreaming is a skill that many children never learn. Yet it has been shown that daydreaming is a skill that not only helps create emotional order by compensating in imagination for unpleasant realities (120), such as the divorce situations described in the previous chapter, but it also helps them:

- rehearse imaginary conditions and circumstances that may bring about good strategies for solving problems
- consider alternative options
- discover unanticipated consequences

These results help increase the possibility of:

- complex thinking
- taking on challenges
- tolerating mistakes and failures
- learning
- happiness

It pays to look at a few cases cited by Mihaly Csikszentmihalyi, who has studied the effects of parental expectations on children. He describes, for example, the child who is pushed by her parents to excel at the violin. The parents may be generally, but not primarily, interested in whether the child is veritably enjoying her playing. They primarily want the youngster to perform well enough to engage an audience, win awards, and end up on the stage of Carnegie Hall. "By doing so, [parents] succeed in perverting music into the opposite of what it was designed to be: they turn it into a source of psychic disorder. Parental expectations for musical *behavior* often create great stress, and sometimes a complete breakdown" (112).

Csikszentmihalyi tells about Lorin Hollander, "who was a child prodigy at the piano and whose perfectionist father played first violin in Toscanini's orchestra. . . . [Lorin] used to get lost in ecstasy when playing the piano alone, but . . . he used to quake in sheer terror when his demanding adult mentors were present. When he was a teenager the fingers of his hands froze during a concert recital, and he could not open his clawed hands for many years thereafter. Some subconscious mechanism below the threshold of his awareness had decided to spare him the constant pain of parental criticism. Now Hollander, recovered from the psychologically induced paralysis, spends much of his time helping other gifted young instrumentalists to enjoy music the way it is meant to be enjoyed" (112).

Before I discuss further the intentions of parents who overschedule their kids, I'd like to prevail once more upon Csikszentmihalyi, who describes the family context that promotes what he describes as *optimal experiences.* He describes such a family as having five characteristics:

> The first one is *clarity*: the teenagers feel that they know what their parents expect from them—feedback in the family interaction are unambiguous. The second is *centering*, or the children's perception that their parents are interested in what they are doing in the present, in their concrete feelings and experiences, rather than being preoccupied with whether they will be getting into a good college or obtaining a well-paying job. Next is the issue of *choice*: children feel that they have possibilities from which to choose, including that of breaking parental rules—as long as they are prepared to face the consequences. The fourth differentiating characteristic is *commitment*, or the trust that allows the child to feel comfortable enough to set aside the shield of his defenses and become unselfconsciously involved in whatever he is interested in. And finally there is *challenge*, or the parents' dedication to provide increasingly complex opportunities for action to their children. (88, 89)

These five conditions: clarity, centering, choice, commitment, and challenge provide "an ideal training for enjoying life" (89). "Children who grow up in family situations that facilitate clarity of goals, feedback, feeling of control, concentration on the task at hand, intrinsic motivation, and challenge will generally have a better chance to order their lives" without exhaustion (89).

Children can have optimal experiences where they feel at liberty to develop their interests that expand themselves without having to argue about rules and controls or worry about their parents' expectations for future achievements and successes. These fortunate kids live in more well-ordered, less chaotic families that parallel those raised with Parental Intelligence, because they have the energy that comes with the feeling of being known as they are and have the implicit parental permission to not be overwhelmed by others' goals.

These kids learn the complexity of enjoying activities scheduled for them and having their own motivations and goals. These are cheerful, happy, strong youngsters who are satisfied with their lives and have strong parent-child bonds. The concept of intrinsic motivation cannot be overemphasized. With Parental Intelligence, parents learn from their children what motivates and interests they have and other activities they can also be motivated to experience for the first time.

I hope it is apparent that I am proposing that children should be challenged and happy; be strong and centered; be emotionally content while highly motivated to explore and discover their interests; and especially *enjoy learning for its own sake.* This is my prescription for parents who employ the Parental Intelligence Way of child-rearing. These are not exhausted kids and they are not overscheduled. They are challenged, enjoy seeking their potential, and are happy.

So why do so many parents—often with their kids' agreements—overschedule their lives like in Lidia's situation in chapter two? These are well-intentioned, devoted parents who want the best for their kids. It is only when these parents face the chaos in their families— the arguing about scheduling, the toll it takes on them when they try to get their rushed kids to their various activities, and ultimately the exhaustion their children feel—that they question their motivations.

They want smart kids. They know the competition their kids will face when they are of college age and want to give them the best preparation for success, however they define it. Perhaps they want their children to have opportunities they didn't have as youngsters, or conversely, perhaps they want their kids to enjoy the same privileges they experienced. Perhaps they want their kids to be more successful than they are, or they want them to be as successful as they perceive themselves to be. These parents generally feel pressured by their adult peers, who follow the same paths preparing their kids for the future, and see their kids' schools encouraging high test scores, superior grades, and participation in the multiple activities they offer.

Some parents do not know that colleges and universities look for kids who demonstrate vested interests in some activities rather than a dazzling array of minimal commitments to diverse choices. Guidance counselors can and do guide these parents and their students to be thoroughly invested in their activity offerings including the arts, athletics, the debate team, school newspapers and magazines, fundraising for valuable causes, political pursuits, and opportunities for leadership.

Schools want to show that they have high acceptance ratings to the top universities, and they encourage elaborate résumé and essay writing in preparation for college applications. The pressures parents put on their kids come, at least in part, from the pressures put on them from their neighbors and school educators. We do indeed live in a competitive world.

Many geographic areas are not as high-pressured as others, and financial resources for education are not the same everywhere. But let's take a hard look at what really makes a kid smart, because international ratings don't put the United States at the top of their lists of achievements in major subjects or in critical thinking abilities. So, something is not working out well for all these dedicated American parents who want high-achieving, happy kids in the long run and instead end up with exhausted children. These parents become discouraged and disillusioned when their plans don't result in the smartest or highest achieving kids in the world.

THE SMARTEST KIDS IN THE WORLD

Despite all of the great intentions of parents in the United States who overschedule their kids hoping to bolster their education and actualize their potential as highly competitive smart kids, it appears—according to a study I shall review—that these students are not only exhausted, but to no avail. There is a great deal of competition in the world for the title *World's Smartest Kids*.

In her book *The Smartest Kids in the World and How They Got That Way* (2013), Amanda Ripley writes:

> Our most privileged teenagers had highly educated parents and attended the richest schools in the world, yet they scored below privileged kids in twenty-seven other nations in math, well below affluent kids in New Zealand, Belgium,

France, and Korea, among other places. The typical child in Beverly Hills performed below average, compared to all kids in Canada. . . . A great education by the standards of suburban America looked, from afar, exceedingly average. (4)

Yet these are the suburban families that overschedule their exhausted children. Something is amiss when "American students score twenty-sixth on a test of critical thinking in math, below average for the developed world" (4). Looking at these results, one might posit that the differences in America versus other countries is our diversity. Also, the United States has a disgraceful child poverty level of about 20 percent, according to Ripley (2013).

Let's compare Norway and Finland, two non-impoverished countries. If poverty and diversity are the source of our problems then what about less-diverse Norway, a welfare state with high taxes, universal health care, and considerable resources. Norwegian children performed just as poorly as our own kids, regardless of their lack of poverty, on an international test of scientific literacy in 2009. By contrast, relatively non-diverse Finland ranked at the top of the world in this question of smartness and solid education. What is extraordinarily noteworthy is that Finland was a place not only where children were loved, which we can presume was common in all these countries, but where *teachers were admired.* Something was amiss in Norway and the US, and it wasn't poverty.

Ripley spent a year traveling around the world and following American exchange students to different countries to learn what was producing the smartest kids. In 2000, a third of a million teens in forty-three countries took a two-hour test called PISA, the Program for International Student Assessment. This test was designed by a think tank called the Organisation for Economic Co-operation and Development, and it measured advanced thinking and communication skills, assessed fluency in collaborative problem solving, and assessed the ability to communicate—all skills that people need to succeed in the modern world.

These skills mentioned above are key features of the steps of the Parental Intelligence Way of approaching child-rearing. Parental Intelligence emphasizes teaching kids critical thinking skills and teaching parents meaning-making, the reasons underlying kids' behaviors and feelings.

Critical skills include:

- empathy
- frustration tolerance
- flexibility

- identifying, clarifying, and expressing ideas
- perspective taking, thinking through the impact of your actions
- weighing options projected into the future and problem solving

PISA promised to make known the measure of teens' abilities to think critically and solve new problems in math, reading, and science, revealing which countries were teaching kids to think for themselves. PISA measured not what kids could memorize but their ability to think creatively.

The number one country in the world on the PISA scoring was Finland, where social background and recession had little impact (see below). While adolescents from the United States did perform better in reading, it was math skills that were expected to predict better future earnings. "In 2009, US teenagers ranked twenty-sixth on the PISA math test, seventeenth in science, and twelfth in reading. We ranked second in the world in just one thing: spending per pupil" (24).

Who was in this large sample of kids isn't specified particularly by Ripley, and more research needs to be done controlling for a wide range of variables, but these results do point us in the direction of questioning what the US parents who are overscheduling their kids want. What are they actually achieving?

It's valuable to look at parent and teacher involvement. Ripley found that the parents of these high achievers "were not necessarily more involved in their children's education, just differently involved" (18). That is, Finnish kids were not noted because they were born smart, but in fact had gotten that way within *a single generation*. Finland was "a system built on trust in which kids achieved higher-order thinking without excessive competition or parental meddling" and these kids did less homework than Americans (24).

Important is that in the single generation, Finland prized the profession of teacher as the US praises the profession of doctor. In fact, getting into the rigorous teacher-training program in Finland was as impressive as getting into medical school in the United States. In the early nineties, when an economic crisis hit Finland with a deep recession and education budgets were cut 15 to 20 percent, national leaders granted a great deal of autonomy to the local Finn educators, who by then "had created their robust system of highly educated, well-trained teachers with high standards. School leaders and teachers were free to write their own lesson plans, engineer experiments within their schools to find out what worked, and generally design a more creative system than any centralized authority ever could" (90).

Ripley points out that parents in Finland "in general seemed to trust their kids more. . . . Teenagers were treated more like adults. There were no regularly sched-uled parent-teacher conferences. None. If teachers had a problem with the student, they usually just met with the student" (98). Parents were not as involved in schools in Finland as they were in the US. These Finnish kids didn't go to after-school tutoring and had more free time than US kids—and not just because they did less homework, but because they were also less likely to play sports or hold down jobs.

On the other hand, parents in Korea—the coun-try that also boasted the highest PISA ratings—were very involved in their kids' educations. In fact, school was the top priority. However, these kids fell asleep in their classes during the day. Their studying took place after school but not in diverse overscheduled activities. Korean parents spent time coaching their kids by read-ing to them, quizzing them, and pushing them to try harder and harder, viewing education as one of their jobs. However, by US standards, many Korean par-ents went too far. Yet they were supported nationally. The day of the big PISA test, the stock market in Korea opened an hour late in order to keep roads free for the students heading to the test, and the taxis gave the kids free rides. Police discouraged people from honking their car horns, so as to not distract students during the English-language listening portion of the test; and airplanes were grounded to limit their noise! In both Korea and Finland—despite their vast differences—kids, parents, and teachers viewed getting an education as serious and more important than sports or self-esteem, according to Ripley's study.

The most unusual part of the Korean education system took place outside of school in what was called a *hagwon*. A hagwon is a private institute that helps kids to cram. At the parents' behest, Korean students became fully engaged at their hagwon. Interestingly, if parents were not fully engaged in their kids' educations, it was considered a failure not of the family but of the hagwon where the parents were customers. The hagwon teachers were free agents who did not have specific certifications; however, their positions were highly competitive because of the expected stellar performance of their teaching methods. "Eight out of ten Korean parents said they felt financial pressure from hagwon tuition costs. Still, they kept paying the fees, convinced that the more they paid, the more their children learned" (174). Ripley termed this whole process as "the country's culture of educational masochism" (174). In fact, competition was so steep that hagwons caught operating past ten o'clock at night by study police were given three warnings, and then they were considered in violation and shut down for a week.

What Finland and Korea held in common was that in these countries learning was intensely important. There was "public respect for learning" (116). The smart kids had specific characteristics as a result: they were rigorous. This meant failure was a part of the learning process that the kids learned to tolerate. Teenagers were expected to manage their own time rather than be dependent on the scheduling of their parents.

Six out of ten of those (exchange students) surveyed said that US parents gave children less freedom than parents abroad. One Finnish student who spent a year in the US pointed out the difference: "In the US, everything was very controlled and supervised. You couldn't even go to the bathroom without a pass. You had to turn all your homework in, but yet you didn't really have to think with your own brain or make any decisions on your own" (117).

Ripley concluded:

> The important distinctions were not about spending or local control or curriculum; none of that mattered much. . . . The fundamental difference was a psychological one. . . . School existed to help students master complex academic material. Other things mattered, too, but nothing mattered as much. . . . The most important difference . . . was the drive of students and

their families. . . . Kids feed off each other. This feedback loop started in kindergarten and just grew more powerful each year, for better and for worse. Schools and parents could amp up student drive through smarter, more meaningful testing that came with real consequences for teenagers' lives; through generous higher grants of autonomy, the kind that involved some risk and some reward; and through quality, more challenging work, directed by the best educated teachers in the world. . . . Those policies were born out of a pervasive belief in rigor. Without it, those things just didn't happen. . . . In the education superpowers, every child knew the importance of an education. . . . In many US schools, however, the priorities were muddled beyond recognition . . . US kids placed a higher priority on sports . . . [which] brought many benefits, including lessons in leadership and persistence, not to mention exercise, but it also brought excessive exhaustion that took away from an academic emphasis. . . . In most US high schools, however, only a minority of students actually played sports . . . and the US obesity rates reflected as much. . . . Valuable life lessons, the ones about leadership and persistence, could be taught through rigorous academic work, too, in ways that were more applicable to the real world. . . . Combined with less rigorous material, higher rates of child poverty, and lower levels of teacher selectivity and training, the glorification of sports chipped away at the academic drive among US kids. (118, 119)

In *The Hurried Child: Growing Up Too Fast Too Soon*, David Elkind compares intense Japanese education to American education. He speaks of the Japanese *juku*, which reminds me of the Korean hagwon in some ways, involving after-school tutoring that goes for several hours each day. Elkind points out that what makes the Japanese education more tolerable is the Japanese mother. Called "Education Mothers" or "Kyoiku Mamas," they are always available for support and encouragement. "Unlike the 'pushy' mother in America—who is often looked down upon with derision—a 'Kyoiku Mama' is looked upon as engaged in a demanding and prestigious profession" (60). However, although the Japanese kids outrank the American kids in math early on, they don't have the same accomplishments at the university level and don't win Nobel prizes voluminously like the Americans. What I find interesting, however, is that Finland's teachers and

Japanese mothers are given a similar high status—a status that we don't necessarily give to teachers and mothers in American life.

Of great importance for what Hadley and Elkind teach, using the Parental Intelligence Way of childrearing supports these characteristics that lead to smart kids. Parents who use Parental Intelligence are involved emotionally with their children and form strong attachments as they reason with them. Children learn the consequences of their behaviors internally, not externally. Parental Intelligence teaches kids persistence and rigor, because this style of parenting demands it by example. Skills learned from parents using Parental Intelligence are directly applicable to the real world because they emphasize critical thinking (flexibility, frustration tolerance, identifying, clarifying and expressing ideas, perspective taking, weighing options projected into the future, and thinking through the impact of your actions on others) and collaborative problem solving in families.

Humanity and rigor in parenting are the keystones of Parental Intelligence that instill an attitude in families that thinking before acting is part of living. It teaches—and then requires—a certain skill set for parents that is transferred to children in their regard for learning in general.

Parents who take the time to use the Parental Intelligence model—and support diligence, conscientiousness, persistence, and thoroughness—more accurately measure achievement. Parents who use Parental Intelligence have high expectations and goals for themselves, as parents who look to collaboratively solve problems in meaningful ways by learning to reason. These skills are regularly conveyed and demonstrated for their children. These parents have a level of self-awareness that they cultivate in their children at young ages. I regard these parents with great prestige, which would indeed parallel the high regard the Korean and Japanese place on their teachers and mothers, respectively. If these high-pressured kids are not exhausted, it's because of the attachment to their parents who support them. In Korea, the kids are exhausted. In Japan, there isn't data from Elkind about that factor.

Getting back to overscheduling, we can see that overscheduling does not necessarily lead to goals of quality achievement, but instead often leads to exhaustion and a lack of intelligent discussion with children about what matters most to them. It doesn't allow parents the time needed to be educational or to be life coaches who read to their children every day when they are small or to talk to them about their days with in-depth conversations as they grow.

Clearly parents have a dramatic impact on their children's lives. But paradoxically, Hadley's research shows that parents who are most active in their kids' schools (such as participating in the PTA) do not necessarily have smarter kids. The impact of your child's education—and thus the impact on his mind—happens mostly at home where parents let their children make mistakes and get back to work. Parents should teach their children how to organize, prize concentration, and give them autonomy.

The five steps of Parental Intelligence—Stepping Back, Self-Reflecting, Understanding Your Child's Mind, Understanding Your Child's Development, and Problem Solving—teach reasoning, understanding, and empathy that allow children to make rigorous problem solving part of their daily lives. These impressive thinking skills that involve executive functioning performed by the prefrontal cortex of the brain involve:

- impulse control
- internalized self-regulation
- organization and the ability to shift between tasks and retain information
- the capacity to focus and attend

The emotional, cognitive, and social processes of working things out build new language and communication skills—often between parents and their children—and form new connections in the brain. These skills are generally built with authority figures, such as when parents help and coach little by little to improve developmental delays with neurocognitive skills. Sometimes parents need this skill training so they can coach their kids. Professionals can enter the picture and help families out, producing short-term resolutions and long-term solutions.

A special kind of exhaustion comes from difficulties with emotion and self-regulation skills. If we consider the critical thinking function noted above, dealing with frustration or other intense emotions, we may notice a child whose emotions go from zero to fifty in a matter of seconds. In his book *Changeable: How Collaborative Problem Solving Changes Lives at Home, at School, and at Work*, J. Stuart Ablon states that "people with poor emotion regulation become 'cognitively debilitated'—they can't think clearly, . . . they fall into severe temper tantrums or episodes of rage, . . . [and they] have a hard time solving problems" (44). If you observe such a person after the tantrum or rage reaction, they are exhausted from the output of so much emotional energy. These people have difficulty mobilizing their cerebral cortex responsible for rational thought and cannot think clearly.

To prevent this cause of eventual emotional exhaustion and needed self-regulation, skills are needed. These skills include:

- thinking rationally, even when upset
- managing irritability, disappointment, and anxiety in an age-appropriate way
- thinking before responding, which includes considering the likelihood of outcomes or consequences for actions
- adjusting one's arousal level to meet the demands of the situation, including waking up after falling asleep (47)

Resolving exhaustion is a complex process for some children and teens with developmental delays in the above skills. This is a problem for parents who don't understand these factors and push for "smart kids." Exhausted children often suffer from being blamed for their misbehaviors, when in fact they lack the skill sets needed for more appropriate behavior.

CHAPTER SIX

BURNOUT AND DEPRESSION

The long history of exhaustion in adults has been looked at medically, socioeconomically, psychologically, and culturally (Schaffner, 2017; Stack, 2008). It is not a modern phenomenon or experience. It is only in children that exhaustion—defined as the depletion of energy—has been neglected; however, it has not been absent in the past. Before child labor laws were instituted in the United States, perhaps there was child and adolescent exhaustion that, although beyond the scope of this book, could be documented.

However, today we are largely discussing the experiences of families who share psycho-social internal and external stressors that lead to exhausted kids. We need to look at the interaction of the mind, body, and society on children. The societal idea that there is something honorable and moralistic in achievement often leads to the burning out of a child. Somehow, this burnout mentality is applauded because of the rigor, persistence, and tenacity of the child who wants to achieve in many areas of life, such as athletics, academics, and the arts. Parents seeking to maximize their children's potential may support this achievement focus, and thus we have the current phenomenon of overscheduling our kids. When a child's life consists of persistent and chronic school stress, the end result is burnout. Lethargy and excessive tiredness are often the complements of loss of enthusiasm and tense nervous energy.

Elkind (2001) purports that "the endless demands for learning in a non-supportive environment and the competition force the young person to call upon energy reserves that are not always replenished. The result (fuel shortage) is exemplified in the child's dissatisfaction with school, fatigue, poor work habits, and sleep disturbances" (193). When in the state of extreme exhaustion, where every reserve of energy has been depleted, we can say that our children have "hit a wall"; similar to a long-distance runner who becomes exhausted and cannot run another step. Elkind speaks of the high school student "who studies so hard for college entrance exams that he or she is too physically spent to take the exams . . . Often [this burnt-out] response is not to the particular set of exams but rather to the accumulated stress of a long history of exam-taking that has taken its toll on the young person's energy reserve" (195, 196).

Parents need to be aware that their children, like themselves, face the danger of depleting limited energy resources and that they may overvalue the supremacy of achievement, as if it was moral and even divine or heroic. Self-discipline is sometimes so overvalued that achievement becomes an obsession, and children are misled into believing that they must be exhaustively competitive and are then superior to others. There is a belief in the virtue of the perpetual battle to overcome weakness that translates to a kind of burnout pride; once again the idea that with physical and emotional work-induced exhaustion, somehow moral superiority is rendered. It presupposes almost a duty of children to achieve exceptionally for their parents. Parents who allow idleness, daydreaming, and being carefree, with this hypothesis, can be viewed as negligent. The result for many adults and children is an inability to relax and replenish one's energy reservoirs—both physically and emotionally—which ironically leads to a lack of:

- productivity
- concentration
- organization
- cognitive and physical achievement

On the other hand, this attitude toward work versus pleasure has also been considered self-exploitation, a kind of masochistic pride in achievement that leads to exhaustion. Being burnt out can lead to disengagement, disillusionment, carelessness, and cynicism about the future, hardly what parents are looking for when they encourage, rather than exploit, their children.

In this book, I carefully consider the needs of each individual; it is important to avoid burnout without leaving physical or mental wounds that impact your children's future aspirations. It is incumbent upon empathic parents not to foist our children too quickly into the adult paradigm of work burnout, a nonmedical diagnosis for potential anxiety and depression.

Schaffner (2017) refers to the "most dominant mind-body metaphor of our times . . . that conceives of the brain as a computer and the body as its hardware." Following this metaphor, our brain can be overloaded and that can lead to a kind of "burnout-related breakdown" (219). Chronic communication and information overload and overstimulation are problems in our increasingly technological society. Interpersonal interactions are reduced to impersonal data exchanges using chronic texting, emails, and computer applications. These can stifle the potential for exploration and conceptualization of deep emotional in-person human responses and reactions. This overload and overstimulation are results of parents viewing their kids from this unhealthy perspective, using the brain as a computer metaphor (Schaffner, 2017). We hardly want our children to turn into exceptional but exhausted robots, depriving them of the pleasures of human contact and the capacity for empathy and critical thinking. Such alienation and disconnectedness could lead to clinical depression.

We must help our children and ourselves find the "off-switch." This switch is needed to prevent the common expressions "running out of steam," "running on empty," "feeling overloaded," "need to unwind" and "recharge my batteries" from becoming part of their everyday language. Theorists have picked up on these metaphors and now think of the human body as a kind of machine that can easily run out of fuel.

Other authors dive deep into how we can enhance our energy resources—which is essential to discover in order for children to lead lives full of creativity and fun!

But first let us look at clinical depression, the sad result for some kids faced with this overachieving standard.

According to the *Diagnostic and Statistical Manual of Mental Disorders, 5th edition* (2013), depression in children can have characteristics that relate to exhaustion. The following depression characteristics are relevant to exhaustion:

- "insomnia or hypersomnia nearly every day" (161)
- "diminished interest or pleasure in activities most of the day, nearly every day" (160)
- "fatigue or loss of energy nearly every day" (161)
- persistent depressive disorder (dysthymia), "a more chronic form of depression that can be diagnosed when the mood disturbance continues . . . for one year in children" (155)

In her book *The Exhaustion Cure* (2008), Stack writes about the impediments of a lack of sleep in children, adolescents, and adults. She is primarily focused on adults, but her good advice can be applied to kids as well. She highlights that "the presence or absence of energy will definitely have an impact on what you're capable of achieving. . . . Energy is the source of productivity" (5). She emphasizes that researchers say an extra sixty to ninety minutes of sleep each night boosts energy levels. Lack of sleep and exhaustion from over activity and over stimulation are related; they can both have the following results:

- decreased performance and alertness
- memory and cognitive impairment
- "interference with carbohydrate metabolism (the breaking down of carbs), which leads to an increase in blood glucose levels, causing insulin to be released, which can lead to weight gain and increased fat storage" (25)

Children who get the proper amount of sleep, which is determined on an individual basis, raise their personal energy level. Thus, burnt-out or depressed kids need to raise their personal energy level in order to achieve well. This information is all imperative for parents as they help schedule activities for their kids; the right amount of activity needs to be a top priority.

Stack's (2008) rule of thumb for the amount of sleep needed is ten to twelve hours for young children and nine hours for teenagers. If a teen sleeps longer on weekends than during the week, this indicates a sleep deficit. With the right amount of sleep, a child or teen will wake up feeling refreshed with energy and will generally not get sleepy during the day. If a child or teen needs to sleep, Stack recommends finishing a nap four to six hours before nighttime sleep. In adults, an hour-long nap provided four times more refreshing sleep than a half-hour nap. It would be interesting to experiment and see if this holds true for children and teens as well.

Another thought to consider it that some children may suffer from seasonal affective disorder (SAD). This is a disorder that occurs when there is a dramatic lack of sunlight—like in the winter months—and it is accompanied by a depressed mood, an energy level drop, often weight gain, fatigue, and difficulty concentrating. Think of it as "their mood merging with the weather." Parents with children and teens affected by SAD need to allow for these possible side-effects, which may cause sleep disturbance, when scheduling activities for their children.

According to Stack (2008), in 1986 the National Institutes of Health discovered that the use of Bluewave technology—an artificial light that is twenty times brighter than natural light—can safely reset one's body clock when used properly (33). The technology can normalize circadian rhythms and improve energy during the day, the ability to fall asleep, and the capacity to awaken more easily (33). It is also important that parents recognize the role nutritional imbalances can play in their children's energy depletion, as the body uses food for repair, growth, and energy. Excessive drug and alcohol usage during adolescence is also very energy depleting.

Oversleeping and exhaustion is common in depression. In chapter three, we saw how Leslie would use sleep to escape from her problems when she was depressed. Exhaustion is common in depressed teenagers and needs to be addressed quickly. Leslie's mother used Parental Intelligence to get at the root of Leslie's difficulties, and together they problem solved how to help Leslie recover. If you want to assess if one of your children is oversleeping, you can consult the National Sleep Foundation and complete the sleepiness test found at this link: https://sleepfoundation.org/quiz /national-sleep-foundation-sleepiness-test.

Stress that overwhelms a person's ability to adapt may also lead to exhaustion. Ordinarily, energy reserves are replenished daily by food and sleep. Generally, parents need to help their kids organize their lives so that their adaptation-energy levels are not depleted when they are stressed. David Elkind (2001) points out in his book, *The Hurried Child: Growing Up Too Fast Too Soon*, that stress is "any unusual demand for adaptation that forces us to call upon our energy reserves over and above that which we ordinarily expend and replenish in the course of a twenty-four hour period" (166). Hans Selye originally created the term *stress response*, or "stress syndrome" or "general adaptation syndrome" (*The Stress of Life*, 1978, xi). *Stress response* occurs when our bodies are called upon to utilize our limited energy reserves. Stress can be positive or negative. Selye (1978) defines negative stress as mental arousal, frustration at one's work or in private life, the necessity of facing responsibilities beyond one's capacities, or physical exhaustion and fatigue (369). He states that "the most important stressors are emotional, especially those causing distress" and that "emotional stimuli with which we are almost constantly faced [can result in] nervous responses (fear, pain, frustration)." The stressor effects depend not so much upon what we do or what happens to us but on the way we take it (370).

Anxiety and worry burn up energy, and this can lead to exhaustion. According to Elkind, children can be stressed by "*responsibility* overload" (171). The issue isn't necessarily how much work is demanded of a child, but the amount of responsibility demanded from a child. Children with too many parental tasks to perform, such as caring for a younger sibling while a single parent is at work, may become stressed by "responsibility overload." Or, a child may go to too many caretakers during a twelve-hour period, which extends her capacity to adapt and sends her into stress overload.

This raises the subject of "*emotional* overload" (Elkind, 172), which is exemplified in *The Busy Parent's Guide to Managing Anger in Children and Teens: The*

Parental Intelligence Way (2018) when two youngsters overhear verbally aggressive arguments between their parents. Overhearing the arguments causes an overload of emotional stress, due to the anger they feel toward their parents—and sometimes each other as a byproduct. Another example is the chronically anxious child who experiences panic attacks or separation anxiety in a rushed household (See Hollman, *The Busy Parent's Guide to Managing Anxiety in Children and Teens: The Parental Intelligence Way* [2018]). The threat of divorce, divorce itself, or parents who travel extensively for work (raising fears the parent will never return) increase separation anxieties in children. These anxieties can exceed their limits to understand and adapt, resulting in emotional exhaustion.

You may recall from chapter one that parents need to understand child development so that their expectations are in-line with the child's developmental stage. If expectancies are too high, the child is stressed and may become exhausted from the pressures he cannot meet.

The stress of "*information overload*" (Elkind, 2001, 181), from the media and technology or from violence in schools, can also exceed a child's capacity to tolerate stress and lead to exhaustion. If there is not time to replenish a child's energy reservoirs with extra sleep after stressful occasions, fatigue is the result. Elkind's point is that children are pushed to grow up too fast—due to these various types of overload—and consequently suffer from stress that they cannot cope with by just additional sleep. Exhaustion will certainly be the result, along with anxiety, depression, and other mental disorders.

Elkind also discusses the fact that children are expected to learn increasingly fast—not only in school but also in summer camps. This hurries them to grow up faster than they are capable of and leads to undue pressures. The rigors of adult competition are hard to keep up with, another source of unending emotional, informational, and physical fatigue. Furthermore, Elkind cites some 500,000 children each year who fly alone—some as young as five years old—due to divorce, travel camps, or training facilities. This is certainly exhausting to our children's emotional resources.

In my work with child-bearing teenagers, I have seen young mothers become exhausted from the physical, emotional, and mental stress of going to high school, completing their homework, and taking care of their babies. "Children's behavior and appearance speak 'adult,' while their feelings cry 'child'" (Elkind, 2001, 12). It seems too often that children are being molded to the needs of adults—adults who are living increasingly pressured, single-parent lives in unsteady work environments with strict scheduling demands—when in fact, the children themselves are suffering. According to Elkind (2001), too many adults are under stress, causing them to lead self-centered lives and to lack the energy needed for dealing with their children's issues apart from their own (27, 28). The Parental Intelligence Way addresses this issue by giving parents an organized, structured plan for parenting that takes both themselves and their children into constant account.

To avoid burnout and symptoms of depression in children, activity and reflection should complement each other. Before investing in a goal, it pays to raise the fundamental questions: Is this something my child really wants to do? Is it something she enjoys doing? Will he enjoy it in the foreseeable future? Is the psychic energy, emotional experience, physical load, and time expended worth it? Do the benefits outweigh the stress load?

According to Selye (1978), indications of stress include general irritability, hyper-excitation, depression, and the predilection to becoming fatigued. Additionally, stress may deprive a child of "joie de vivre" and lead to insomnia, which is usually a consequence of being "keyed up" (174, 175). Children and teens need to be encouraged by their parents to find out what they intrinsically want. Learning for its own sake as well as for future achievements need to be considered. Teaching our children to pay attention to their goals is as important as the activities themselves.

Parents and kids shouldn't be so wrapped up in external goals that they fail to work together. Playing with these ideas could be enjoyable and exhilarating for children and their parents. Child and parents can use the planning time to get to know each other in ways that they haven't before. Not only can the children discover and explore what they want to learn at different life stages, but parents can be self-reflecting on their hopes and dreams for their children. Try to master the ability to make these journeys into thoughts and feelings about what your child desires and hopes for. This teaches your child to internalize the capacity for lifelong assessments; once learned, these skills will benefit them as they grow into adulthood.

According to Csikszentmihalyi (1990), "If goals are well chosen, and if we have the courage to abide by them despite opposition, we shall be so focused on the actions and events around us that we won't have the time to be unhappy" (227).

It is remarkable for kids when their parents prize their *intrinsic* motivations and thinking. That is, when parents acknowledge that their children have genuine interests, desires, and challenges that they can discover within themselves, it results in satisfying feelings of accomplishment and hopes for many future opportunities. This is the task of step three of Parental Intelligence: understanding your child's mind.

A further gain of the Parental Intelligence Way is the increase of the art of conversation within a family. Csikszentmihalyi (1990) exclaims that "the main function of conversation is not to get things accomplished, but to improve the quality of experience" (129). With conversations, parents and their children create a world of words that not only passes on information but creates new ideas. Conversation among parents and their children gives children the experience of being recognized as existing in their own right, affirming their sense of self. "Even one word" from parent to child "is enough to open a window on a new view of the world, to start the mind on an inner journey" (131). Such gratifying and creative experiences improve the quality of both parent's and children's lives—without exhaustion!

CHAPTER SEVEN

THE IMPORTANCE OF PLAY

*A*ll work and no play are certainly harmful at any age, but what is work and what is play for each individual child? According to Selye (1978) and following our discussion about stress in the previous chapters, "If there is too much stress in the body as a whole, you must rest" (416). He goes on to say that we need work, but it must be diversified. That is, deviation in work is important in combating mental stress. For example, nothing is accomplished by telling worriers not to worry; however, a remedy may be found in telling worriers to put their thoughts in a different direction or diversion (419).

Unconditional acceptance is particularly important to children. When parents threaten to withdraw their love from a child when she fails to measure up, her natural playfulness will be gradually replaced by exhaustion. This is because of the waning of adaptive resources due to stress and chronic anxiety. When a child's brain is adapted for an environment of chaos, threat, and distress, he is ill-suited for the playground and enjoying the intrinsic value of learning for its own sake.

What is the importance of play for children and adolescents? Play is a way of communicating concerns and needs and expressing oneself. It can be done through playing with characters, drawing, imagining stories, or any other creative method that resonates with the child. Resonating with the child's sense of self is a key element in play, as compared to an activity that weighs on the child due to the intensity of the parents' goals for their child. Ideally and on average, adults work for eight hours each day; sleep for another eight; and then eat, relax, and play for the remaining eight. In a society that hurries children's development beyond its natural course, we find that play is minimized. Healthy self-love is restorative, and genuine play can be seen as that kind of self-love.

Children need to be given the opportunity for pure play as well as work. Fantasies such as fairy tales help children deal with the conflicts of life. Free play where children imagine and use toy figures to act out ways of dealing with challenges enhances their development. It gives them an opportunity to deal with the stresses of life. Playing with real things, like baking a cake, gives children the feeling of coping with reality under plea- surable interactions with others, including peers and adults. These different forms of play give children the feeling they have some control over their own destiny. They begin to trust in their own resources. They are not self-centered but experiencing unself-conscious assur- ance, which leads to trust in oneself.

The "autotelic self" translates potential threats into enjoyable challenges (Csikszentmihalyi, 1990, 209), and children do this through play.

The term literally means a

> self that has self-contained goals, and it reflects
> the idea that such an individual has relatively
> few goals that do not originate from within the
> self. [The child] knows that it is she who has
> chosen whatever goal she is pursuing. What
> she does is not random, nor is it the result of
> outside determining forces. . . . Knowing them
> to be her own, she can more easily modify her

goals whenever the reasons for preserving them no longer make sense. In that respect an autotelic person's behavior is both more consistent and more flexible. (209, 210)

This a highly sophisticated view of play where the autotelic child concentrates and can sustain involvement. It is through their themes and characters and plots that kids explain their thoughts and feelings. Self-consciousness is not a diversion or a problem unless a parent interferes. Each child, instead of worrying about how she is doing or looks from the outside, is wholeheartedly committed to her goals. This is what Csikszentmihalyi describes as a "flow" experience that gives meaning to life. Children can do this through play. They can shift entropy or exhaustion into a challenge to obtain vitality and meaning, finding order from disorder in their daily experiences and thus in their own minds.

As discussed in earlier chapters of this book, the United States is falling behind other countries in academic fields. Some explanations are: the focus on excess screen time, test-driven curricula, adult-driven childhood sports, and the near elimination of creative and playful teaching. Rote learning often replaces critical, innovative thinking.

Love, work, and play come together to enhance all age levels. Looking at child development, infants by twelve months learn object permanence: an object not seen, still exists. This results in children playfully looking for and retrieving hidden objects over and over, mastering this new learning experience. The toddler who drops his food off his high chair for his mother to retrieve it may annoy his mother, but he is having a grand time proving his object permanence knowledge—over and over. Further, he is proving that what goes away can be found and retrieved. This knowledge grows into hide-and-seek, for example, as three-year-old children learn object constancy and practice the appearance and disappearance of loved ones. Play, love, and work are thus interwoven as the child grows.

By ages two to six, play becomes quite dominant through self-created learning experiences with themes of lost and found, dependence and independence, distrust and trust. During the elementary school years, ages six to twelve, children become industrious. They adapt to the demands of a social world where school is a primary focus, but play cannot be left behind. Play themes continue to become more complex as the child dramatizes herself or her toy figures as the one in authority, reversing the roles of the real world by making believe she is the teacher, mother, fire chief, and burglar. Through these reversals, the child feels more powerful and self-assured in daily life. Passive turns into active, and identification with the aggressor is revealed in improvised play.

In a local private school near my home, the curriculum is project based. Whatever interests the children becomes the curriculum around which reading, writing, and arithmetic are learned. The children love school, because it is not differentiated from play but is filled with discovery and exploration. The discovery method in math and science with manipulative tools is of far more interest to children than rote learning.

By ages eight to twelve, games with rules are fascinating to kids, especially as their peers are more interesting playmates and buddies than adults are. When playing with other children, the rules often change to suit their needs, but everyone soon learns that the same rules must be applied to all the players consistently. These children also play by ordering their world with collections of various objects that strike their fancy. These are not exhausted children; they are vibrant and active with seemingly ceaseless energy.

In early adolescence, love interests begin to be revealed with the advent of puberty. Play is the way to interact with peers, and a way to turn away from parents and toward social companions for fun and mutual engagement. Art and music are means of expressing feelings and conflicts, and it is often best for parents not to interfere but to nonjudgmentally acknowledge their teen's creativity. Fantasy play is replaced with fantasy novels. One example is *Harry Potter*, with themes of loss and recovery, life and death, cunning and prejudice, friendship, rivalry, teamwork and loyalty, good and evil, leadership and heroism, and magic and power. Others are *The Hobbit* and *Lord of the Rings* trilogy, where good and evil reign again; violence and peace are explored; friendship and fellowship triumph; enemies and loyalties abound; and the small empathic hobbits become the larger than life heroes. Romance novels are also popular, where social themes are played out; and favorite books about wimpy kids and nerds who explore, discover, and overcome obstacles become widespread.

By late adolescence, play, love, and work are all interwoven once again. Play becomes more complex and structured, in the form of the arts and athletics, in preparation for future career goals.

In this age of newer and newer technology, children learn to use computer-driven games with great skill at earlier ages. Their knowledge of symbols is encouraged with the icons on their well-known games. Children become the experts and their parents the students. This enthusiasm for educational video games does not bring a loss of the imaginary play that children invent for themselves. It is an addition—contrary to the beliefs of many naysayers who fear the innovative toys of today. Some building toys like LEGO seem timeless; younger and younger children fill this marketing niche, creating far more advanced vehicles and buildings than the instructions suggest—all with little LEGO people socializing in their midst as they are solving problems.

Too much screen time with television can be a hindrance to time spent reading and being read to, but reading is dictated by the parents' love for reading, and parents should model a love of reading for their children.

Children who are playing are not exhausted children. They are happy and cheerful, exploring and discovering fun for learning and fun for its own sake. They build forts out of pillows on a couch and wood and limbs in their yards. They climb trees to prove their strength and prowess and race around, expending the wonderful energy of their youth.

One great remedy for the exhausted, stressed-out child is self-initiated and self-directed play—uninterrupted by parental interpretation and guidance. If parents hover and redirect play because they think more is being learned, the child can be come disinterested, bored, and exhausted from the stress of interference. They are being taught that their play is not of value. It is an art to think like children and play at their intended pace. Being more of an observer on the sidelines is often the best role for parents who want to understand how their kids play and *how they view the world differently than adults.*

HOW FANTASY PLAY HELPS THE EXHAUSTED CHILD

The intensity and intentionality of children's play will easily convince an adult of its importance. In my office is a simply built dollhouse with two floors and a big drawer below. This drawer is a surprise to most young kids; it is the basement. The roof comes off and I have various simple pieces of furniture, toilets, sinks, and dolls of different shapes and sizes. In my office I also have blocks of varying sizes; plastic animals, soldiers, boats, and cars; stuffed animals and puppets; and dress-up clothes. Further, I have crayons, colored pencils, and markers to use with plain white paper, both standard size and huge rolls.

The most frequently used object for boys and girls alike, up until about age nine, is the dollhouse, where children invent stories of varying lengths to express themselves in any way they see fit. The second most popular choice is a large set of large, colorful, soft blocks of different shapes and sizes. The third most popular choice is drawing.

Why do the children take these choices over the more defined toys? Simply because with these, they can make up their own stories and narratives that express their pleasures, worries, problems, questions, and reasons for feeling exhausted. In my thirty years of practice, no child has become exhausted from playing in my room. They may come in exhausted (or their parents report their exhaustion), but their inventive play never tires them out. In fact, playing is a remedy for mastering daily stressors and exhaustion.

Here are some brief examples. One little six-year-old played primarily with my blocks for about a year. She came in to the session overtired and left with vitality. Each time she built a new village or singular house. The theme was constant: because her family members were unclear, she was looking for a home that was safe and contained. Her father, who was not married to her mother, came and went unpredictably until the end of treatment. By then, his disappearances had been addressed and he came to live in the household with the mother, whom she eventually married. When it was time to end the treatment, the little girl was displeased until she learned she could visit me any time she wanted. She hasn't yet; she just needed to hear that I wouldn't disappear.

A selectively mute five-year-old girl played consistently with the dollhouse. Her chronic theme was a mother doll kidnapping a tired baby and throwing her out the window. This child began to talk to me and only me for many months. At first, she spoke in short phrases and then in full sentences. She was being given permission to direct her own play, which was about a depressed mother and alienated father who were soon to separate. She feared for her security and couldn't talk, for fear of being punished for her feelings of anger and anxiety. Sadly, when she began to talk at home, her parents ended the treatment. They felt my work was done when it was just beginning. Hopefully, the child's feelings were allowed as this small family came apart at the seams.

A ten-year-old girl always talked quietly on a chair about questions she had, like a little adult. Then she drew consistently perfect looking girls just like herself in expensive pretty outfits with well-designed hairstyles. She was exhausted in large part from what gave her rest, the bed: only problem was, it wasn't hers, but her parents. She had been sleeping in their bed nightly since she was a baby. The parents were professionals who worked long hours, and the little girl and her parents missed each other during the day and after school, when she stayed with her alcoholic grandmother. This little girl had no friends. She was always tired, because she and her parents never got enough rest. In time, her perfectionistic standards were relaxed, and she learned to sleep in her own bed, made friends, and discontinued treatment successfully. Her questions and drawings revealed the perfectionism in her mind and home and some obsessive qualities that needed to be understood. She learned she could express playfully aggressive thoughts and feelings and that they were part of life. This liberated her from her perfectionistic standards and gave her a child-like life.

A three-year-old boy was overtired and raced from object to object, having trouble settling down. He finally collapsed by the big blocks and made them into a long tunnel that he could fit through. He went inside one end and out the other—over and over. The tunnel contained him emotionally and made him feel safe. It also showed him that if he disappeared, he would reappear each time he made his journey, and I would be there. His parents both worked different shifts: his mother during the day; his father during the night. He was never sure of where they were and when they would be together next, because it was rare. Later, the tunnel became a car wash, and he was the car that was all cleaned up by the end of his tunnel journey. His tiredness and upset feelings were washed away, because he had found a vehicle to regulate his emotions. Eventually his father came to play with him, and he showed him this game. The father cheered each time his son came out of the car wash, reinforcing the boy's safety and regularity in a predictable fashion. This boy returned for treatment years later, as a young teenager, after his parents separated.

I won't forget six-year-old Ari who was in the midst of a messy divorce. He came in dutifully twice each week, driven by a chauffeur. I would find him sitting patiently alone in the waiting room. He was always on time. He would walk in and immediately get on the floor and mew like a kitten. He would then take the cushions off the couch, put them in a circle, and get inside like it was a nest. In a short time, he invited me in as the mommy cat, and we rested together. This exhausted child found his place of peace by his own imagination and by the means at his disposal. Years later he returned as an adult who was living with a friend in an apartment, wanting to verbalize his continued struggle with his coworkers. It was soon discovered that these adults represented his parents; in different ways, they were causing him problems in performing for them, although he had developed excellent abilities in his career by this time. Remarkably he was also still having arguments with his mother about how to raise and take care of their many cats. Fortunately, he had learned to talk directly to his mother about how he felt he wasn't taken care of by her in his youth. Even though, he still displaced these conflicts onto other adults in his life, like his coworkers.

Luckily, he was wise enough to see that he wasn't viewing the conflicts clearly and that he needed to sort it all out. Even with his higher-level cognitive capacities, he still trusted in me; trust sustained all those years that had begun with his fantasy play and rich imagination.

These examples show that—regardless of sophisticated toys and screen time—when given the opportunity, children play using their own resources: the ideas and feelings in their minds. They play actively in narratives that reveal their troubles and pleasures. They do not need to be taught to play; they just need the time to do so. In an overscheduled world of school and activities, this can be undervalued. Learning is enhanced by play. Critical thinking is developed in the stories children enact with their figures and themselves. Flexibility; empathy; understanding the impact of their actions on others; toleration of frustration and disappointment; overcoming obstacles and mistakes, successes and failures; and goal-driven activities and problem solving begin to take place more and more as they mature.

THE EFFECTS AND BENEFITS OF PLAY ON BRAIN STRUCTURE AND FUNCTIONING

When play enhances curiosity, it encourages memory and learning. Play helps kids deal with stress, such as life transitions. High amounts of play are associated with low levels of cortisol, and play activates norepinephrine at synapses, which facilitates learning and improves brain plasticity. Cortisol is a steroid hormone that regulates a range of processes throughout the body—when provided in the right amounts, it supports the immune response and metabolism. It is also very important in helping the body respond to stress. With nurturance, caregiving "may indirectly affect brain functioning by modulating or buffering adversity and by reducing toxic stress to levels that are more compatible with coping and resilience" (Garner et al., 2018, 5–6).

Play encourages executive functioning, which is a focus on how we learn rather than the content of what we learn. There are benefits in cognitive flexibility, inhibitory control, and working memory—all of which enhance sustained attention and the elimination of distracting details, as well as better self-regulation or self-control and problem solving. With improved executive functioning because of play, impulsiveness, emotionality, and aggression regulated by the amygdala in the brain are minimized.

Peer play influences the ability to learn to negotiate, to problem solve rules of a game, and cooperation. For example, particularly with low-income children, when preschool kids are given blocks to play with at home with minimal adult direction, they show language improvements at a six-month follow-up. Similarly, kids in active play for one hour a day were more able to think creatively and multitask. Pretend play enhances the ability to collaborate and reason about hypothetical results.

Further, there are health benefits of play that involve physical activity, such as promoting healthy weight and cardiovascular fitness and strengthening the immune and endocrine systems. And most pertinent to this study of child exhaustion, play decreases stress, fatigue, njury, and depression, while increasing range of motion, coordination, balance, and flexibility. Of interest is that kids pay more attention to class lessons after free play at recess than after structured physical education programs, which may point to increased activity during their free play (Garner et al., 2018, 7).

In conclusion, the American Academy of Pediatrics points out that kids need a variety of skill sets in order to heighten their development and manage toxic stress (Garner et al., 2018). If left without these skill sets, their stress has a higher likelihood of leading to exhaustion, a state of extreme physical or mental fatigue. The Academy's research demonstrates that developmentally appropriate play with peers and parents is an opportunity to promote healthy social, emotional, and cognitive development.

Voluntary play is spontaneous and fun. It builds executive functioning skills and school readiness, creating an imaginative reality of pretending. Play goes beyond just having fun to include taking risks, testing boundaries, and experimenting. Learning thrives when children are given control over their actions through play; that is, they feel a sense of agency when they have a role in their own learning, as new skills scaffold on previous skills. Kids who play are like little scientists, learning as they look and listen to their peers around them (Garner et al., 2018).

CHAPTER EIGHT

THE SCIENCE OF SLEEP AND EXHAUSTION

NORMAL SLEEP IN CHILDREN AND ADOLESCENTS

United States population studies show that approximately 30 percent of preschoolers and between 50 percent and 90 percent of school-age children and adolescents do not get as much sleep as they may need. The pervasive use of screen-based media is a potential contributor to widespread sleep insufficiency. Screen-based media devices are present in the bedrooms of 75 percent of children, and around 60 percent of adolescents report viewing or interacting with screens in the hour before bedtime. In a recent systematic review of 67 studies of screen time and media use in school-age youth and teenagers (1999–2014), 90 percent of the research found that screen time was adversely associated with sleep health, primarily via delayed bedtimes and reduced sleep duration. Potential mechanisms underlying these observations include: (a) time displacement (i.e., time spent on screens replaces time spent doing other things, including sleep); (b) psychological stimulation based on media content; and (c) the effects of light emitted from devices on circadian timing, sleep physiology, and alertness. Healthy sleep patterns in childhood and adolescence suggest a lower obesity risk, better psychological well-being, improved cognitive functioning, and a decrease in risk-taking behaviors. Sleep among children and adolescents should be a priority in the family (LeBourgeois et al., "Digital Media and Sleep in Childhood and Adolescence," 2017).

Thus, sleep duration decreases substantially from infancy through adolescence, with increased sleep in adolescence at the nighttime period only. Although the development of sleep is a dramatic and relatively rapid process during the first decades of life, changes in sleep continue across the life-span (McLaughlin, C. et al., *Dev. of Neuroscience*, 2009).

THE STAGES OF SLEEP
REM versus Non-REM Sleep

The brain is sometimes more active when a person is asleep than when he is awake. Scientists once thought that sleep was a passive state, a time when a person's brain and body shut down for the night to rest and recover. But now, researchers know that sleep is a highly active time, a period during which the brain and some physiological processes may be hard at work. For example, some hormones involved in childhood growth, cell repair, and digestion are improved during sleep. Brain pathways involved in learning and memory also increase, according to the National Institutes of Health (NIH). But sleep can also slow down many other physiological processes, from heart rate and breathing to body temperature and blood pressure. The stage of sleep a person is in affects how active the brain and body are (Nierenberg, *Live Science*, 2017).

For more than sixty years, sleep researchers have known that there are two major categories of sleep:

REM sleep, which stands for "rapid eye movement," and non-REM or non–rapid eye movement sleep (Dr. Stuart Quan, clinical director of the division of sleep and circadian disorders at Brigham and Women's Hospital, Boston, MA, in Nierenberg, *Live Science*, 2017).

According to Quan, non-REM sleep consists of three stages, known as N1, N2, and N3. Before 2007, non-REM sleep was broken down into four stages, but then sleep medicine specialists decided that there was no physiological reason to distinguish between two of the stages, the old stage three and stage four sleep. Those were combined into one stage, now referred to as N3. During sleep, the brain repeatedly cycles through these four distinct stages—REM and the three non-REM stages—of sleep in a specific sequence. This sequence changes somewhat between the first and second half of sleep. As sleep progresses through a series of four to five sleep cycles, the time spent in the REM stage gets longer and the time spent in N3 sleep gets shorter.

Non-REM Sleep

Stage N1

When a person gets drowsy, she is drifting into N1 sleep. In this first stage of non-REM sleep, a person is making the transition from being awake to falling asleep. This is a relatively light form of sleep that lasts about five to ten minutes. During this stage, heart and breathing rates begin to slow, eye movements also slow, and muscles relax. Body temperature decreases, and brain waves, if observed on an electroencephalogram (EEG) in a sleep lab, would be seen to slow.

A person can be easily awakened from N1 sleep and may not think she has actually slept. N1 sleep is the first stage entered when taking a nap. It's normal for a person to experience "hypnic jerks," also known as "sleep starts," during N1 sleep. These are sudden, brief muscle jerks that may happen with a falling sensation. When the hypnic jerks occur, the sudden movements may or may not wake the sleeper up. Adults spend the least amount of time in stage N1 sleep, which represents about 5 percent of their total sleep time.

Stage N2

Shortly after N1 sleep ends, a person enters this second stage of non-REM sleep, which typically lasts ten to twenty-five minutes (Quan, in Nierenberg, *Live Science*, 2017). Stage N2 sleep is also considered a period of light sleep. During this stage, eye movement stops, heart rate slows, brain waves become slower, and muscles relax even further.

As night progresses, a person spends more time in stage N2 sleep than in any other sleep stage, according to the National Institutes of Health. Adults spend about 55 percent of their total sleep time in stage N2 sleep.

Stage N3

Non-REM sleep then progresses into its third stage, which is often referred to as "slow-wave," "delta," or "deep" sleep. (Delta waves are a type of slow brain wave typically seen during this stage on EEG in a sleep lab.)

N3 sleep is a period of deep sleep that is needed for an individual to feel refreshed for the next day. A person typically spends more time in the N3 stage during the first half of sleep than the second half, but why is still a mystery. Typically lasting twenty to forty minutes, N3 sleep is when the brain becomes less responsive to external stimuli, and as a result, it is most difficult to wake a person up from this stage. Someone awakened from N3 sleep is extremely groggy and disoriented, which is why people may not want to nap for more than thirty minutes.

During N3 sleep, heart rate and breathing slow to their lowest levels. Blood pressure falls slightly, and body temperatures drop even lower. Muscle activity decreases, and there is no eye movement.

This is also the stage when sleepwalking and sleep talking are most likely to occur. "Nightmares and night terrors are also N3 sleep phenomenon," Quan said.

(Night terrors, also called sleep terrors, typically occur in children and involve a child sitting up in bed during sleep and screaming, according to the Mayo Clinic.)

Slow-wave sleep occurs for longer stretches in babies and young children, and the time spent in N3 sleep decreases steadily with age for reasons that are unclear. According to Quan, adults typically spend about 15 percent of their total sleep time in stage N3.

REM Sleep

A person first enters REM sleep about ninety minutes after falling asleep, having gone through all three stages of non-REM sleep. The first REM cycle of the night typically lasts about ten minutes, but each subsequent REM stage gets progressively longer as the night goes on. The characteristic sign of REM sleep is that a person's eyes move rapidly from side to side beneath closed eyelids. However, this eye movement is not constantly occurring. Scientists don't know exactly why rapid eye movement occurs during REM sleep, although some have hypothesized that it's linked with dreaming.

Supporting that idea, REM sleep is the stage when most dreaming and vivid imagery occurs (Quan, in Nierenberg, *Live Science*, 2017).

People often don't remember much of their dreams, but they are more likely to recall some aspects of a dream if awakened from REM sleep. During this kind of sleep, heart rate climbs and blood pressure rises slightly compared with N1 sleep. Body temperature falls to its lowest point during sleep. Arm and leg muscles deeply relax to the point of being almost immobile, possibly to prevent people from acting out their dreams, according to the Mayo Clinic.

Breathing becomes fast and shallow, and the brain may be even more active during this stage of sleep than during wakefulness, sleep experts say. REM sleep is when the brain processes information from the day so that it can be stored in long-term memory, according to the National Sleep Foundation.

CHILD'S SLEEP HABITS

According to the US National Library of Medicine National Institutes of Health, parents reported that children ages six to seventeen years old typically spent 9.3 hours in bed on school days and 10.2 hours on non-school days. Parents also estimated how much sleep their child obtained at night. Approximately 45 percent of all children obtained ≥9 hours of sleep per night on school nights, and 69 percent of all children slept ≥9 hours on non-school nights. Shorter sleep duration was more common among older children: more than half (56 percent) of fifteen- to seventeen-year-olds slept ≤7 hours per night, and only 10 percent slept ≥9 hours. Among six- to eleven-year-olds, 8 percent slept ≤7 hours per night, and 23 percent slept only 8 hours per night (*Sleep Health*, 2015, 15–27).

As we have seen, sleep in infants and children is highest but declines and levels off in adolescence and adulthood. Amounts of the individual sleep stages change as well. REM sleep percentage is high in infants and children, declines until adolescence, then remains relatively constant during adulthood. Slow-wave sleep is also highest in infants and children, declining slowly after adolescence. A decline in sleep in children was noted during school days. Generally speaking, total amount of sleep per day declines by the age of two and continues to drop to about eight hours a day in the second decade of life.

During slow-wave sleep, children sleep deeply: it takes a loud sound or other stimuli to awaken them. EEG activity is slowly making its appearance until it is well developed by about age eight when it may occur.

There are childhood sleep disturbances, such as sleep apnea, that manifest themselves in behavioral disturbances during waking hours, including behaviors similar to ADHD, aggressiveness, or excessive shyness. To help with these sleep disturbances, the removal of tonsils is often the most beneficial procedure. However these disorders, as well as nightmares and night terrors, are common in children as well as some adolescents.

With night terrors, the child lets out a loud scream and displays fear and signs of autonomic arousal, such as a rapid heart rate and respiration. The child is usually not aroused easily, is not consolable, and doesn't report dreams, but ultimately returns to sleep with no memory of the event in the morning. These events typically occur in the first half of the night. Sleep apnea and restless legs may also be problems that affect a child's sleep. Be aware that there is a strong genetic component to these disorders. Sleep terror management includes making sure the child is not sleep deprived and that daytime sources of anxiety or stress are addressed. Naps can be helpful, as well as finding scheduled awake times that are usually associated with the nightmares had during REM sleep and perhaps unwittingly associated to the disturbing dreams involving fear, anger, or disgust. These nightmares more likely to occur in the second half of the night and—contrary to sleep terrors—are usually remembered. Nightmares, a REM sleep phenomenon, fit in the second half of the night when REM is more plentiful. Relationship difficulties or other sensitivities may be common in those with chronic nightmares (Mendelson, W. B., 2017).

Snoring occurs in roughly 7 percent of children, most frequently when they're lying on their backs. Other sleep disorders—such as restlessness during sleep—are more common in people over forty but may occur in children. Turning throughout the night may occur. In contrast, some children periodically have very specific, discrete movements of the limbs, known as periodic limb movement disorder. This involves a very brief flexion of the hip, knee, and ankle, lasting five to ten seconds and occurring about every twenty to forty seconds (Mendelson, W. B., 2017). And of course, excessive sleepiness due to lifestyle deprivation may also occur—due to excessive overscheduling of children, as discussed earlier.

Narcolepsy-cataplexy affects both boys and girls and typically appears between the ages of ten and twenty, although about one-quarter of the cases begin after age twenty. Nearly two-thirds of those with narcolepsy have cataplexy, which means they have type 1 narcolepsy. Cataplexy is the sudden and brief loss of muscle strength or muscle tone brought on by strong emotions or situations such as laughter, surprise, and stress. For those with narcolepsy-cataplexy, sleepiness and falling asleep may occur during the day. Childhood onset is associated with the increased likelihood of being overweight or developing premature puberty, as it increases the release of sex hormones. Depressed mood may also be an accompaniment.

Another common occurrence might be micro-sleep. This is when children fall asleep from one to ten seconds during the day. Unfortunately, episodes of micro-sleep may lead to incidents of memory loss. Of course, there are other conditions that cause excessive sleepiness in children, including insufficient sleep, sleepiness due to medicines or medical conditions, and menstrual-related hypersomnia.

SLEEP DEPRIVATION AMONG ADOLESCENTS

Sleep deprivation among adolescents is *epidemic*. This is due in part to pubertal changes in the homeostatic and circadian regulation of sleep during the teenage years. These changes promote a delayed sleep phase that is exacerbated by evening light exposure and incompatible with features of modern society, such as early school start times (Hagenauer et al., *Dev Neurosci*, 2009).

A recent poll by the National Sleep Foundation found that over 45 percent of adolescents in the United States obtain inadequate sleep. At the root of this chronic sleep deprivation is the adolescent tendency to stay up late. Teenagers maintain later bedtimes than younger adolescents, even when wake up times are constrained by school or work. This delayed timing of sleep is popularly attributed to many external influences, ranging from work to social opportunities. Current evidence demonstrates, however, that social factors as well as physiological underpinnings account for the adolescent delayed sleep onset. Girls begin to show a delay in the timing of sleep, meaning they fall asleep at a later time one year earlier than boys, paralleling their earlier pubertal onset. These sleep differences between girls and boys may be due to a sexual differentiation itself, or it may be due to a masking of the exhaustion phenomenon by the estrogenic rhythms around the time of ovulation.

Adolescents continue to show a delayed circadian (or internal clock) phase, as indicated by daily endocrine rhythms, even after several weeks of regulated schedules that allow for enough sleep. This delay is even maintained under controlled laboratory conditions in which there is limited possibility for social influence. Both home-based and laboratory studies of adolescents show that the delayed circadian phase correlates with secondary-sex development (puberty)—if we assume that teenagers attending the same grade in school are exposed to a similar social environment.

The Kleine-Levin syndrome, another sleep disorder seen particularly in male adolescents, consists of long periods of sleepiness with a fluctuating course and is often accompanied by binge eating, an increased sex drive, and a depressed mood (Mendelson, 2017, 127).

THE MECHANISM UNDERLYING ADOLESCENT CHANGES IN SLEEP PATTERNS

There is a natural tendency for adolescents to have a "phase delay"; that is, both the beginning and the end of their sleep shifts to a later time. Such later sleep times occur before the onset of puberty and conflict with the need to get up for a school that begins at 8:30 a.m. or earlier. Additionally, the need for sleep may increase during older adolescent years, having effects that result in chronic sleep deprivation and a potential impact on information retention.

On weekends, younger teens tend to sleep in about the same amount, but older teens often sleep in one or one and a half hours later. Since the older teens usually go to bed even later on weekend nights, the result for the week as a whole is an irregular sleep pattern. This all makes adolescents predisposed to sleep disorders. Teens with later bedtimes during the weekdays are more likely to have an increased body mass index, compared to others with the same amounts of sleep and exercise.

Girls report being awake longer before falling asleep, but then sleep longer than do boys. This may be due to the onset of menstruation for those who develop insomnia. Boys who develop insomnia are inclined to do so at an earlier age (Mendelson, 2017, 92, 93).

Initially, in adolescence slow-wave sleep is high, like in childhood. Early teens may miss their first REM period because of the large amount of slow-wave sleep. Later, as the percentage of slow-wave sleep declines, REM seems to come earlier in the sleep cycle. This adolescent decline in slow-wave sleep is striking in the sleep EEG—it may drop by 50 percent between ages ten and twenty. The slow-wave sleep decline usually occurs earlier in girls than in boys and seems to correlate with the progressive degree of sexual maturation. Another interesting aspect of slow-wave sleep decline is that it is part of a major reorganization of the brain during adolescence when there is a decline in the number of interconnections between cortical neurons, decreased plasticity of the brain, and initiation of more adult thinking processes (Mendelson, W. B., 2017, 93).

Traditionally, the timing of sleep is thought to derive from two primary endogenous components: a circadian timing system (sleep-wake cycle) and a homeostatic drive (maintenance of internal stability despite environmental changes). The homeostatic drive for sleep—or sleep pressure—increases with the duration of waking and dissipates during sleep. In humans, the circadian timing system promotes wakefulness in the evening and promotes sleep in the early morning. Adolescents develop a resistance to sleep that permits them to stay up later. At the same time, their circadian phase becomes relatively delayed, which provides them with a drive to stay awake later in the evening and to sleep later in the morning.

ADOLESCENT CHANGES IN THE HOMEOSTATIC DRIVE TO SLEEP

Homeostasis is the tendency of the human body to maintain internal stability and balance, compensating for environmental changes. Only a few cross-sectional studies have examined homeostatic sleep drive in adolescents. One study of extended wakefulness in early-, pre-, and post-pubertal teens tested for sleep propensity at two-hour intervals. Data showed that more mature adolescents are slower to fall asleep at critical times (after 14.5 and 16.5 hours awake—i.e., in the late evening), relative to younger adolescents. These findings indicate that more mature adolescents are able to tolerate somewhat longer waking episodes than pre-pubertal adolescents. This supports the growing conjecture that the circadian period and the light sensitivity of the circadian system are altered during puberty. Such changes could explain the development of a delayed slow-wave sleep phase during puberty.

SLEEP AND MEMORY IN HEALTHY CHILDREN AND ADOLESCENTS

There is evidence that sleep is important for learning, memory, and the underlying neural networks. Most studies support the hypothesis that sleep facilitates working memory as well as memory links. There is also evidence that performance in abstract and complex tasks that involve higher brain functions declines more strongly after sleep deprivation than performance in simple memory tasks. Future studies are needed to better understand the impact of a variety of variables potentially modifying the interplay between sleep and memory, such as developmental stage, socioeconomics, circadian factors, or the level of post-learning sensory and motor activity (Kopasz et al., *Sleep Medicine Reviews*, June 2010, 167–177).

THE INFLUENCE OF SLEEP QUALITY, SLEEP DURATION, AND SLEEPINESS ON SCHOOL PERFORMANCE IN CHILDREN AND ADOLESCENTS

Insufficient sleep, poor sleep quality, and sleepiness are common problems for learning and memory in children and adolescents. The associations between sleep quality (N = 13,631), sleep duration (N = 15,199), sleepiness, (N = 19,530) and school performance were examined in three separate meta-analyses that included influential factors (e.g., gender, age, parameter assessment) as moderators.

All three sleep variables were statistically significant but modestly related to school performance. Sleepiness showed the strongest relation to school performance, followed by sleep quality and sleep duration. Effect sizes were larger for studies including younger participants, which can be explained by dramatic prefrontal cortex changes during early adolescence. Concerning the relationship between sleep duration and school performance, age effects were even larger in studies that included more boys than in studies that included more girls, demonstrating the importance of the different pubertal development of boys and girls (Dewald et. al, *Sleep Medicine Reviews*, June 2010).

DIGITAL MEDIA USE AND SLEEP IN SCHOOL-AGE CHILDREN AND ADOLESCENTS

A recent review shows a consistent association between media and sleep in children and adolescents ages five to seventeen from diverse geographic regions around the world. Over five dozen observational studies using cross-sectional approaches have examined associations between screen time (i.e., television, computer, video games, mobile devices) and a variety of sleep parameters. In over 90 percent of these studies, more screen time was associated with delayed bedtimes and a shorter total sleep time among children and adolescents. Computer use was more consistently associated with poor sleep outcomes than television was, perhaps because watching the television may be less interactive than computer-based activities. Among studies on the association between television use and sleep timing and/or quality, over 75 percent found links between television use and insufficient sleep.

In a recent cross-sectional study of a representative sample of children (six to seventeen years of age) in the United States, whether or not technology (e.g., phone, computer, TV) was left on overnight in the child's bedroom was a significant predictor of insufficient, age-appropriate sleep duration.

Although it was found that the majority of studies observed a relationship between tiredness and television viewing, computer use, video game play, or mobile phone use in children and adolescents, the effects of media exposure on tiredness may be age dependent. For example, media use in adults has been associated with sleep onset latency but not with tiredness—as adults who spend a substantial amount of time engaging with media may have the opportunity to compensate by sleeping longer. Such a compensatory mechanism is largely impossible for children and adolescents, as their wake times are primarily determined by parents, school hours, and/or extracurricular activities. This suggests that future research should address links between digital media use and sleep between weekdays and weekends, as well as between school term and holidays.

New technologies, digital platforms, intrusive/engaging software, and media-related behaviors are rapidly changing, and we still don't have a complete understanding of their impact on sleep and health. Data from a recent cross-sectional study of 454 adolescents found that more than 60 percent of youth kept their mobile phones with them when they went to bed, and more than 45 percent used their phone as an alarm. This reflects the high prevalence of digital media in the sleep spaces of adolescents. Furthermore, a recent study of approximately 2,000 fourth and seventh graders indicated that sleeping near what was defined as "a small screen" was associated with increased tiredness. Among US children and adolescents, poorer sleep quality is associated with leaving technology on overnight in the bedroom.

THE INFLUENCE OF LIGHT ON CIRCADIAN PHYSIOLOGY AND SLEEP HEALTH

Finally, we do not know the extent to which the effects of digital media on sleep affect and/or amplify other aspects of child health and development. Sleep has not been fully incorporated into studies investigating the effects of media on other outcomes. In particular, little is known about developmentally-based susceptibilities to digital media and associated exposure to bright LED-based screens.

The recent American Academy of Pediatrics policy statements about media use in children and adolescents reports the following sleep-related recommendations:

- Talk with families about the importance of sleep and healthy sleep expectations.
- Encourage a bedtime routine that includes calming activities and avoids electronic media use.

- Encourage families to remove all electronic media from their child or teen's bedroom, including TVs, video games, computers, tablets, and cell phones.
- Talk with families about the negative consequences of bright light in the evening on sleep.
- If the child or adolescent in your care is exhibiting mood or behavioral problems, consider insufficient sleep as a contributing factor.

SLEEP IN PSYCHIATRIC ILLNESS: DEPRESSION AND ANXIETY DISORDERS

Less than three decades ago depression was seen as a predominantly adult disorder: children were considered too developmentally immature to experience depressive disorders, and adolescent low mood was seen as part of "normal" teenage mood swings. Developmental studies have been central in modifying that view. Few would now doubt the reality of child and adolescent depressive disorders, or that youth depression is associated with a range of adverse outcomes, including social and educational impairments as well as both physical and mental health problems later in life. In addition, however, while research on the course and correlation of depression has identified important similarities across development, it has also highlighted age-related variations; as a result, investigators continue to evaluate the extent to which childhood, adolescent, and adult onset depressions reflect the same underlying condition.

Given this prevalence of depression in children and adolescents, sleep—or the lack thereof—has arisen as an important factor. Insomnia is prevalent in those with troubled minds. Difficulty sleeping occurs not only in depression but also in panic disorders. Further, insomnia is a risk for later developing depression. Research has shown that continued insomnia is a risk for later suicide and is accompanied with reported feelings of hopelessness. Thus, it may be that insomnia leads to depression and/or is characteristic of depression.

Of interest, it may also be that partial sleep deprivation is being used to reduce depression, especially when the child has traumatic memories that may be present during sleep through nightmares. Some children or adolescents may be prolonging sleep in order to avoid reliving their trauma in sleep (Mendelson, W. B., 2007, 138, 139).

Sleep during depression is generally short, shallow, and fragmented, with REM sleep occurring early with intense eye movements. This is generally more true in unipolar depression, as a bipolar illness is more likely to be accompanied by excessive sleepiness. When sleep is short, shallow, and fragmented, total sleep time is generally reduced, with many awakenings during the night. Classically, clinical histories of those with depression reveal that depressed people awaken early in the morning, that they are then unable to go back to sleep, and that the sleep they get is shallow. In other words, during depression there is a reduced amount of slow-wave sleep. Furthermore, depressed youngsters experience a shorter amount of time between the onset of sleep and the first REM period. In non-depressed people, the first REM period of the night is relatively brief, with subsequent ones getting progressively longer. For those who are depressed, in contrast, the first REM period is relatively long, so that there is not a progression in length as the night goes on (Mendelson, W. B., 2007, 136).

Anxiety disorders are found to be the most common mental health disturbance experienced by youth. Sleep-related problems (SRPs) are highly prevalent among anxious youth and encompass a variety of problems, including nighttime fears, insomnia, and refusal to sleep alone. Chronic sleep disturbance is associated with a range of behavioral and physical problems in youth and predicts future psychopathology. One study investigated the relationship between sleep problems and anxiety sensitivity in a sample of 101 anxious youth, ages six to seventeen. Heightened anxiety sensitivity significantly predicted prolonged sleep onset latency (delayed sleep onset) across the sample, even after accounting for severity of anxiety, depression, and age (Weiner et al., *Journal of Anxiety Disorders*, 2015).

CONCLUSIONS

Children generally have better age-appropriate sleep in the presence of household rules and regular sleep-wake routines. Sufficient sleep quantity and adequate sleep quality were protected by well-established rules of sleep hygiene (limited caffeine and regular bedtimes). In contrast, sleep deficiency was more likely to be present when parents and children had electronic devices on in the bedroom after bedtime. Public health intervention goals for sleep health might focus on reducing the encroachment of technology and media into bedtime and supporting well-known sleep hygiene.

An important consequence of our modern-day, 24/7 society is that it is difficult for families—children and caregivers both—to get adequate sleep. Sleep in the family context involves reciprocal interactions between all members of a household, interactions with the environment of the home, and external factors affecting any member. Several potential reasons include the use of technology in the bedroom; complicated and busy daily schedules with competing work, school, social, and recreational activities; neighborhood noise from vehicular traffic, commercial, or industrial activity; neighbors; and psychiatric disorders.

In the 2014 Sleep in America Poll sponsored and funded by the National Sleep Foundation (www.sleep foundation.org), the majority of parents endorsed the importance of sleep for health and well-being. Parents placed great value in the importance of sleep—both for their own health and well-being and for their child's health and well-being. Despite this, most children in this sample (nearly 90 percent) obtained less sleep than currently recommended and less than what has been observed across many countries and developmental groups. Parent-reported child sleep duration varied with age, with younger children (six to eleven years of age) sleeping longer than adolescents (twelve to seventeen years of age). In this sample of US households, parents and their children generally reported better age-appropriate levels of sleep in the presence of household rules and routines regarding sleep. Sleep deficiency was more likely to be present when parents and children did not adhere to sleep hygiene standards, such as not leaving engaging electronic and media devices on in the bedroom.

It is not just a matter of obtaining sufficient sleep quantity—children and adolescents, like adults, also need adequate sleep quality.

For policy makers, teachers, and parents, these results provide a clear mandate. The effects of sleep deprivation on grades, car accident risk, and mood are indisputable (Hagenauer et al., *Dev Neurosci*, 2009). A number of school districts have moved middle and high school start times later, with the goal of decreasing teenage sleep deprivation. Results indicate that later school start times lead to decreased truancy and drop-out rates. We can also help teenagers gain control over their own sleep patterns by teaching sleep and circadian principles in middle and high school health education. Minimizing exposure to light at night, as well as reducing computer or TV usage immediately before bed-time, can naturally advance circadian phases. Similarly, incorporating outdoor morning activity into a teenage schedule can reduce trouble falling asleep at night.

The Advantages of the Parental Intelligence Way

The use of the Parental Intelligence approach to solving exhaustion problems in children and adolescents is helpful. Discussing with children their sleep habits in a non-blaming, nonjudgmental way interests them in solving their sleep problems significantly. This approach is empathic and instructive for kids because it takes away the punitive association many kids have with bedtimes from a young age. Understanding what is on your child's mind about their sleep patterns helps parents problem solve with them how to get enough sleep. Children are curious and interested in sleep science as it affects their daily life and are thus rather easily engaged in discussions about their afternoon naps and evening sleep patterns. The Parental Intelligence Way is a boon to sleep science knowledge among kids and a great way to resolve sleep onset and delay problems. In using Parental Intelligence with the information in this book, you will be well on your way to helping your child get enough sleep each night and, thus, function productively and happily during the daytime hours.

REFERENCES

Ablon, J. Stuart (2018), *Changeable: How Collaborative Problem Solving Changes Lives at Home, at School, and at Work*, TarcherPerigee, New York.

American Academy of Pediatrics, *Pediatrics*. March 2012, Vol. 129, Issue 3.

American Psychiatric Association, *Diagnostic and Statistical Manual of Mental Disorders* 5th ed. (2013), Arlington, VA: American Psychiatric Association.

Carpenter, Siri, American Psychological Association, *Monitor* Staff, October 2001, Vol. 32, No. 9 Print version: page 42 (/monitor/oct01/index.aspx).

Child Adolesc Psychiatr Clin N Am., 2009 Oct. 18(4):799–811.

Csikszentmihalyi, Mihaly, (1990), *Flow: The Psychology of Optimal Experience*, Harper and Row, New York.

Dewald, Julia F., Meijer, Anne M., Oort, Frans J., Kerkhof, Gerard A., Bögels, Susan M., The influence of sleep quality, sleep duration and sleepiness on school performance in children and adolescents: A meta-analytic review, *Sleep Medicine Reviews*, Volume 14, Issue 3, June 2010, pp. 179–189; https://di.org/10.1016/j.smrv.2009.10.004.

Elkind, David (2001), *The Hurried Child: Growing Up Too Fast Too Soon*, 3rd ed., Da Capo Press, Cambridge, Mass.

Findley, Dr. Sheri M. (Jan 2008) *Paediatrics & Child Health* (13(1), pp. 37–42).

Garner, A., Hutchinson, J., Hirsh-Pasek, K., Yogman, M., Michnick Golinkoff, R. (2018), The Power of Play: A Pediatric Role in Enhancing Development in Young Children, American Academy of Pediatrics Clinical Report, *Pediatrics*, Volume 142, Issue 3, https://doi.org/10.1542/peds.2018-2058.

Hagenauer, M.H., Perryman, J.I., Lee, T.M., and Carskadon, M.A., Adolescent changes in the homeostatic and circadian regulation of sleep, *Dev Neurosci.* 2009, 31(4):276–84. doi: 10.1159/000216538. Epub 2009 Jun 17.

Hollman, Laurie (2016), The Exhausted Child, *Pittsburgh Parent Magazine*, Pittsburgh, PA. http://www.pittsburghparent.com/Pittsburgh-Parent /Web-2016/The-Exhausted-Child/.

Hollman, Laurie (2015), *Unlocking Parental Intelligence: Finding Meaning in Your Child's Behavior*, Familius, Sanger, Calif.

Hollman, Laurie (2018), *The Busy Parent's Guide to Managing Anxiety in Children and Teens: The Parental Intelligence Way*, Familius, Sanger, Calif.

Hollman, Laurie (2018), *The Busy Parent's Guide to Managing Anger in Children and Teens: The Parental Intelligence Way*, Familius, Sanger, Calif.

Kaufman, J., Martin, A., King, R.A., Charnery, D., Are child, adolescent, and adult onset depression one and the same disorder? *Biol. Psychiatry*, 2001, June 15, 49 (12): pp. 980–1001.

Kopasz, Marta, Loessl, Barbara, Hornyuak, Magdolna, Riemann, Dieter, Nissen, Christoph, Piosczyk, Hannah, Voderholzer, Ulrich, Sleep and memory in children and adolescents—A critical review, *Sleep Medicine Reviews*, Volume 14, Issue 3, June, 2010, pp. 167–177. https: doi.org/10.1016/j.smrv.2009 .10.006.

LeBourgeois, M.K., Hale, L., et al., Digital Media and Sleep in Childhood and Adolescence. *Pediatrics*, 2017 Nov; 140 (Suppl 2): S92–S96.

McLaughlin, Crabtree V., Williams, N.A. (2009). *Dev Neurosci.* Jun; 31(4): 276–284. Published online 2009 Jun 17.

Mendelson, Wallace B. (2017), *The Science of Sleep: What It Is, How It Works, and Why It Matters*, The University of Chicago Press, Chicago, Ill.

Nierenberg, Cari, REM vs. Non-REM Sleep: The Stages of Sleep, *Live Science*, July 19, 2017, *Pediatrics*, 2017 Nov; 140 (Suppl 2): S92–S96.

Ripley, Amanda (2013), *The Smartest Kids in the World and How They Got That Way*, Simon and Schuster, New York.

Schaffner, Anna Katharina (2017), *Exhaustion: A History.* Columbia University Press, New York.

Selye, Hans (1978), *The Stress of Life*, rev. ed., McGraw-Hill, New York.

Stack, Laura (2008), *The Exhaustion Cure: Up Your Energy from Low to Go in 21 Days*, Basic Books, New York.

Weiner, C., Ekins, M., Pincus, D., Comer, J., Anxiety, sensitivity and sleep-related problems in anxious youth, *Journal of Anxiety Disorders* 32, May 2015, pp. 66–72.

RESOURCES

National Sleep Foundation: Children and Sleep: https://sleepfoundation.org/sleep-topics/children-and-sleep.

National Sleep Foundation Sleepiness Test: https://sleepfoundation.org/quiz/national-sleep-foundation-sleepiness-test.

Adolescent Changes in the Homeostatic and Circadian Regulation of Sleep. M.H. Hagenauer, J.I. Perryman, T.M. Lee, M.A. Carskadon: https://www.ncbi.nlm.nih.gov/pmc/articles/pmc2820578/#R70.

The Science of Sleeping in Childhood: https://www.sleepio.com/articles/parent-sleep/the-science-of-sleeping-in-childhood.

www.sleepfoundation.org.

ABOUT THE AUTHOR

LAURIE HOLLMAN, PhD, is a psychoanalyst with specialized clinical training in infant-parent, child, adolescent, and adult psychotherapy. She specializes in modern parent-child relationships and is an award-winning, three-time author. She has been on the faculties of New York University and the Society for Psychoanalytic Training and Research, among others. She has written extensively on parenting for various publications, including the *Psychoanalytic Study of the Child*, *The International Journal of Infant Observation*, *The Inner World of the Mother*, *Newsday's Parents & Children Magazine*, and *Long Island Parent* in New York. She blogged for *Huffington Post* and currently blogs for *Thrive Global*. She also writes for *Active Family Magazine* in San Francisco and is a parenting expert for *Good Housekeeping* and *Bustle Lifestyle*. Her Mom's Choice Award winning books are: *Unlocking Parental Intelligence: Finding Meaning in Your Child's Behavior*; *The Busy Parent's Guide to Managing Anxiety in Children and Teens: The Parental Intelligence Way*; and *The Busy Parent's Guide to Managing Anger in Children and Teens: The Parental Intelligence Way*. She has also recently written *The Busy Parent's Guide to Managing Technology with Children and Teens* and *Are You Living with a Narcissist? How Narcissistic Men Impact Your Happiness, How to Identify Them, and How to Avoid Raising One.* Learn more on lauriehollmanphd.com.

She is married with two spirited adult sons.

ABOUT FAMILIUS

Visit Our Website: www.familius.com

Join Our Family

There are lots of ways to connect with us! Subscribe to our newsletters at www.familius.com to receive uplifting daily inspiration, essays from our Pater Familius, a free ebook every month, and the first word on special discounts and Familius news.

Get Bulk Discounts

If you feel a few friends and family might benefit from what you've read, let us know and we'll be happy to provide you with quantity discounts. Simply email us at orders@familius.com.

Connect

- Facebook: www.facebook.com/paterfamilius
- Twitter: @familiustalk, @paterfamilius1
- Pinterest: www.pinterest.com/familius
- Instagram: @familiustalk

The most important work you ever do will be within the walls of your own home.

CPSIA information can be obtained
at www.ICGtesting.com
Printed in the USA
JSHW020709230420
5219JS00005B/6